BASICS OF AUDIOLOGY

From Vibrations to Sounds

BASICS OF AUDIOLOGY

From Vibrations to Sounds

JERRY L. CRANFORD, PhD, MCD, CCC-A

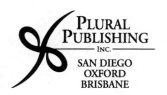

PLURAL
PUBLISHING
INC.
SAN DIEGO
OXFORD
BRISBANE

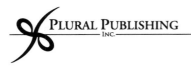

5521 Ruffin Road
San Diego, CA 92123

e-mail: info@pluralpublishing.com
Website: http://www.pluralpublishing.com

Typeset in 10½/13 Palatino by Flanagan's Publishing Services, Inc.
Printed in the United States of America by Edwards Brothers Malloy
19 18 17 16   5 6 7 8

Library of Congress Cataloging-in-Publication Data

Cranford, Jerry.
  Basics of audiology / Jerry Cranford.
      p. ; cm.
  Includes bibliographical references.
  ISBN-13: 978-1-59756-180-8 (pbk.)
  ISBN-10: 1-59756-180-0 (pbk.)
  1. Deaf—Rehabilitation. 2. Audiology. 3. Hearing disorders—Diagnosis.
  [DNLM: 1. Hearing Tests—methods. 2. Audiology. 3. Auditory Diseases,
Central—diagnosis. 4. Hearing—physiology. 5. Hearing Disorders—diagnosis.
WV 272 C891b 2007] I. Title.
  RF297.C7365 2007
  617.8—dc22

                                                                    2007010321

Contents

Preface

For many years, audiology (AUD) and speech-language pathology (SLP) have been closely interdependent health care entities. Many years ago, when the two disciplines were newer and had smaller and less complicated databases and scopes of practice, some students pursued combined graduate training and clinical certification in both areas. In the past two or three decades, both disciplines have rapidly expanded to the point that it is now very difficult for students to specialize in more than one area. However, because of the close professional interdependence of the two fields, students pursuing doctoral degrees in audiology (the Doctor of Audiology or Au.D. degree, which in 2007 will replace the master's degree as the entry level requirement for clinical practice) must take basic courses in the speech and language areas, while students pursuing degrees in SLP must take courses to acquire a solid basic understanding of audiology. In terms of traditional educational jargon, students need to "major" in one area and "minor" in the other area.

Fortunately, minoring requires less classroom and clinical practicum training than does majoring in an area. The author is an American Speech-Language-Hearing Association (ASHA) certified clinical audiologist (Certificate of Clinical Competency awarded 1985) and long-time hearing scientist (Ph.D. awarded in 1969) who yielded to his faculty's "SOS" for someone to develop and teach an introductory audiology course to groups of "non-background" SLP graduate students who had limited undergraduate coursework in the field of audiology and all of its basic science precursors (acoustics, anatomy and physiology of the ear and nervous system, and psychoacoustics). Unfortunately, the author is not aware of any textbook that has been written specifically for this subgroup of students. Most students who enter graduate training programs in speech-language pathology have had undergraduate training in speech and hearing. Students with undergraduate backgrounds typically begin their graduate training with more advanced clinical audiology courses that assume solid prerequisite knowledge in the basic science background areas. However, many speech-language pathology graduate training programs also accept highly motivated students (i.e., with high Graduate Record Examination scores) with no undergraduate training in these prerequisite areas. The present text has been written specifically for these non-background students. It assumes little or no prior knowledge of the basic or clinical sciences that underlie the field of audiology.

In addition to being useful in undergraduate training programs as a primary or supplementary text, a book of this type could also be valuable for SLPs who have been "in the trenches" for a number of years and who feel they need to have their knowledge of audiology refreshed or updated. Since the author has focused on using nontechnical or layman's terminology in explaining the various scientific and clinical concepts/principles in this field, he also believes that parents, relatives, or significant others of patients with hearing impairments might also find this book useful for understanding the problems experienced by their loved ones.

References and Suggestions for Further Reading

For readers who want to know more about the profession of audiology, the author recommends the following two excellent sources:

Martin, F. N., & Clark, J. G. (2006). The profession of audiology. *Introduction to audiology* (9th ed.). Boston: Allyn and Bacon.

Stach, B. A. (1998). The profession of audiology in the United States. *Clinical audiology: An introduction.* San Diego, CA: Singular.

PART

I

The Scientific Background for Audiology

Audiology is a practical clinical branch of the basic science field of psychoacoustics (the psychology or perception of the physical or acoustical properties of sound), which in turn is a branch of the larger discipline of psychophysics (the psychology or perception of all physical stimuli, including vision, hearing, somatosensory or touch, olfactory or smell, etc.). As a distinct clinical discipline, audiology is a neophyte compared to other biomedical fields, having emerged following World War II when returning veterans across the country began flooding Veterans Administration Hospitals complaining of severe hearing losses incurred during the war. As a practicing speech and language pathologist (SLP), the student will need to acquire a solid understanding of the essential scientific background for the profession of audiology, as well as a working knowledge of what audiologists do and what important information they can provide to assist in the management of their patients. The SLP professional will not be required to learn how to perform the different test procedures used by audiologists, but they must be able to communicate with people and understand the various written audiological evaluation reports the audiologist may send or the patient may bring to the SLP clinic.

In the following chapters, the author will describe and explain the basic scientific information that SLPs must acquire in order to understand what the audiologist may convey to them in verbal or written reports. The specific science areas that will be covered include physics of sound or acoustics, functional anatomy/physiology of the peripheral and central parts of the auditory nervous system, and psychoacoustics. All three of these scientific disciplines are very extensive and complex, and even those who pursue PhD academic/research degrees in each area cannot possibly learn everything about them. Those who pursue clinical doctoral degrees in audiology must also have extensive knowledge of the three areas, but they do not need to learn as much as required for the PhD degree. As practicing SLPs, students will need to know a significant amount about these fields, but they can relax knowing that it will not be necessary to learn as much as their audiology classmates. The author will only describe the essential information that the SLP professional will need to assist in understanding the hearing status of patients. The author promises, as much as possible, to limit the use of technical jargon, although it will be necessary to cover the specialized terminology that the audiologist may use in communications with SLP colleagues.

CHAPTER

1

Physics of Sound or Acoustics

In order to understand how the ear transforms vibratory energy from the environment into nerve impulses that are used by the higher centers of the brain to allow perception of sounds, the student must understand what sound is. All physical objects in the universe are made up of matter, in the form of atoms (the basic building blocks), molecules (collections of atoms), and more complex structural entities (pinnae, eardrums, middle ear ossicles, etc.). The amount of matter in a given object determines the object's density. Denser objects contain more atoms per unit volume than less dense objects. The least dense objects in the universe are interstellar regions of space that, although not a total vacuum, do contain very small numbers of atoms per unit volume (star dust?). The densest objects in the universe are the so-called "black holes." These are large stars that have collapsed onto themselves to the point that they are extremely dense and have gravitational fields that are so strong that light cannot escape and, ergo, they cannot be seen. If the matter in black holes could be weighed, a piece of matter the size of the tip of your little finger would weigh more than a Navy aircraft carrier.

Different types of matter have different densities and for our purposes can be thought of as differing in stiffness. Denser objects (also sometimes referred to as having more mass or being more massive) tend to be stiffer and more resistant to being moved (or

3

stopped, when already moving) by externally applied forces. Another formal term used by physicists for this property of matter is elasticity. This refers to the ability of an object to bounce back to its original shape after being compressed (bent or deformed) by an external force. The more elastic or stiff an object, the more readily it will return to its original shape after being deformed. All objects will begin to vibrate if a sudden external force (like a hammer blow) is applied. The object will continue to vibrate until some external force makes it stop, such as its rubbing against adjacent objects. All objects, regardless of their density, size, and so on, can be made to vibrate. In this text, we will keep things simple and only discuss the vibration of objects that are directly related to human hearing, such as air molecules, eardrums, middle ear ossicles, earphones, and loudspeakers. Water molecules can be made to vibrate and you can hear when your head is underwater. Steel can also vibrate, and folklore has it that Native Americans used to put their ears on the railroad tracks to detect the white man's approaching trains long before they could be seen.

Almost every textbook on the subject of acoustics has introduced the subject of sound using the analogy of the vibrating tuning fork (Figure 1–1). Tuning forks were originally invented by musicians to allow the accurate tuning of stringed musical instruments, such as guitars and pianos. For many years, otolaryngologists used tuning forks to evaluate certain aspects of their patients' hearing (many still do). Because numerous textbooks contain excellent descriptions of tuning forks and how they can be made to produce *pure tones* of different *frequencies*, which are known as *sine waves*, the author will only summarize the basic elements of these descriptions that directly apply to how we hear airborne sounds and how airborne sounds physically interact with the physical structures of the ear (either normal, injured, or diseased) to modify the final acoustic stimuli that are sent to the brain for processing.

Tuning forks come in all sizes and shapes, but are typically designed to have a very specific range of densities and stiffness. When struck by a hammer (or the heel of the examiner's shoe), the tines of the fork will begin to vibrate at a specific rate, which is dependent on the specific density (stiffness) of the tuning fork. Denser or stiffer forks will vibrate faster, whereas less stiff forks will vibrate at slower rates. The back-and-forth movement (vibration) of each tine will alternately push and pull away from the surrounding

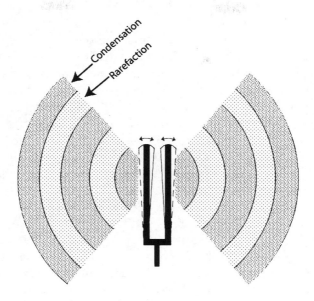

Figure 1–1. Shows the regions of condensation (increased air pressure, air molecules bunched closer together) and rarefaction (decreased air pressure, air molecules further apart) that occur when the tines of a tuning fork vibrate back and forth after being struck (e.g., by a hammer or the heel of a shoe). In reality the alternating regions of rarefaction and condensation radiate in all directions away from the fork in the form of an expanding sphere.

air molecules to produce small regions of denser air (more molecules per unit volume) that alternate with less dense regions (fewer molecules per unit volume). As the tines continue to move to and fro, these regions of higher density (known as regions of condensation) continue to alternate with lower density regions (regions of rarefaction). Figure 1–1 depicts this effect. It is important to note that it is the regions of condensation and rarefaction, and not the air molecules, which travel away from the source of the vibration (tines). The analogy of dropping a rock in a pond of still water to create ripples spreading outward is frequently used in textbooks on acoustics. Another analogy is termed the *domino effect* and involves setting a large number of closely adjacent dominoes upright on their ends and then pushing the first one over. This starts a chain of events in which each domino as it falls causes the next domino to fall. While the individual dominoes stay in place, it is the "falling action" that moves down the row of dominoes. The differing rates of vibration produced by tuning forks with different densities is referred to as the frequency of the pure tone. This rate of vibration or frequency is measured in hertz (abbreviated as Hz) or sometimes as cycles per second (abbreviated as cps). If the tuning fork vibrates more quickly, it will have a higher cps or Hz value. If it vibrates more slowly, it will have a lower cps or Hz value. One complete cycle involves the tines moving inward from their undisturbed neutral starting point to produce an adjacent region of rarefaction and then moving outward to produce a region of condensation and then back to the original neutral starting point. The analogy of a swinging pendulum (with an ink pen attached to the bottom) hanging directly above a moving strip of paper can be used to depict the traveling waves (air pressure changes) that move away from the sound source (Figure 1–2A). As the pendulum swings back and forth (to simulate the inward and outward movements of the tuning fork tines), the paper continually moves from right to left below the moving pen. The movement of the pen on the paper produces a regularly repeating wavelike tracing that depicts the traveling sound wave (Figure 1–2B). In terms of trigonometry, the term *sine wave* is often used to describe those waves that vibrate at a constant and fixed rate. Your author will refrain from going any further into this physical/mathematical analogy, although he would recommend interested students might consult more advanced textbooks to clarify their understanding of this phenomenon.

The different textbook descriptions of tuning forks, pure tones (sine waves), regions of condensation or rarefaction, and the like, while useful for understanding the basic properties of simple sounds, do not convey enough information to fully understand the nature of complex sounds (e.g., speech sounds), which is more what we clinically oriented folks need to know about. While atoms are the building blocks of physical objects, pure tones or sine waves are the basic building blocks of complex sounds. To understand how the ear and brain process the more frequently encountered complex sounds, we must also understand the important concepts of natural resonant frequency and how sounds physically interact with other objects (walls, ceilings, chairs, etc., as well as the different physical structures of the ear, such as pinna, ear canal, eardrum, etc.) in terms of transmission (i.e., transferring vibrating energy from one

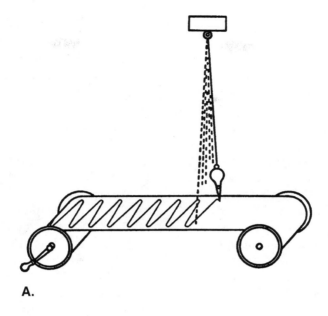

A.

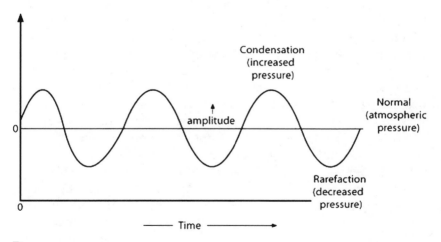

B.

Figure 1–2. Pure tones, or sine waves, are the basic building blocks of all complex sounds. They occur very rarely in the natural environment. Shown in this figure are the physical characteristics that hearing scientists or acoustic engineers use to formally describe or define this type of sound. (**A**) Depicts the analogy of a swinging pendulum (containing a pen) drawing a sinusoidal tracing on a moving strip of paper. (**B**) Defines the different components of the sine wave in terms of underlying changes in amplitude and air pressure over time.

medium, like air, water, etc., to another) or reflection (that is, vibratory energy being reflected away from the surface of one medium, like a wall, into another medium, such as air). Most sounds are complex and so are the physical structures (both outside and inside the head) that they have to interact with before becoming the neural impulses in the brain that allow us to perceive the sounds. Figure 1–3 shows examples of how multiple simple sine waves can be combined to produce more complex waveforms. Hearing scientists (and some audiologists) have access to special tools (electronic equipment) for "dissecting" a complex waveform into its basic building blocks (sine wave components). This technology is called Fast Fourier Transformation (FFT). This process allows us to take any complex waveform and identify the frequency and amplitude of each of its pure tone components, as shown in Figure 1–3.

All physical objects (tuning forks, your skull, the diaphragm of a loudspeaker, etc.), if disturbed by another object (a hammer blow, an electric current), will begin to vibrate. This vibration will continue at the same rate until some adjacent object(s) causes the vibration to "dampen" or grow weaker and stop. Damping occurs when the vibratory energy of the object (tuning fork) is completely transmitted to adjacent objects (surrounding air molecules). All objects, depending on their specific density and stiffness (and elasticity), possess what is termed a *natural resonant frequency*, which is a rate (frequency) at which they will vibrate with the least amount of externally applied energy. For example, a tuning fork with a specific density/stiffness will begin to vibrate at a specific frequency when struck once by a hammer. This rate of vibration is referred to as the natural resonant frequency of this particular tuning fork. Because it was struck only once by the hammer, this vibration is referred to as *free* or *unforced vibration*. It is also possible to force the tuning fork to vibrate at a faster or slower rate or frequency by continually applying the external force (e.g., hammer blows) at another specific rate. This is referred to as forced vibration and is the usual way in which sounds are created. During speech, the human vocal cords are being continually bombarded by external forces (e.g., flowing air from the lungs plus muscle contractions triggered by higher neural centers) to create the complex speech sounds that consist of hundreds of different sine waves continually changing in amplitude and frequency in a complex fashion. A loudspeaker when playing music is also being bombarded by changing forces (in this case, electrical cur-

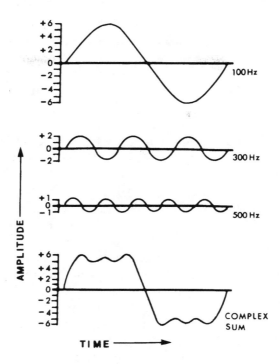

Figure 1–3. An example of a complex waveform. The top three wave-forms (with frequencies of 100, 300, and 500 Hz) are the pure tones or sine waves that make up the complex waveform shown in the bottom waveform (complex sum). Whenever complex waveforms are created, the regions of condensation and rarefaction that move away from the sound source become very complex, as does the pattern of vibration on the basilar membrane of the cochlea. The individual regions of condensation and rarefaction created by each individual pure tone component interact with the regions of condensation and rarefaction created by the other pure tones. The different regions may physically add or subtract from each other to produce a very complex pattern of air molecule movements. (Reprinted with permission from *Speech Science Primer* (2nd ed.) by G. Borden and K. Harris, 1984, Baltimore: Williams & Wilkins.)

rents), which can be visualized as a multitude of sine waves continually changing in frequency and amplitude (the strength of the vibration). Some of these forced sine waves are closer to the natural resonant frequency of the loudspeaker and require little additional externally applied energy to vibrate at this frequency. More energy is required to force the particular loudspeaker to vibrate at frequencies that are further from its natural resonant frequency. When any object is forced to vibrate at frequencies that are different from its natural resonant frequency, some distortion will occur. Distortion consists of other frequencies being created that are different from the natural resonant frequency of the object. These distortion products are typically higher in frequency than the object's natural resonant frequency and are referred to as *harmonic overtones* (because they are even multiples of the original tone).

The difference in density or stiffness between woofers and tweeters is why the former are best suited to play low frequency components of music and the latter high frequency sounds. This natural resonant frequency phenomenon also explains why women, whose vocal cords tend to be stiffer, have higher fundamental voice frequencies than men. This physical explanation of why less externally applied force is required to cause objects to vibrate at their "preferred" natural resonant frequencies can also explain some other natural phenomena that the reader has no doubt noticed in daily life. A glass of water will often shatter when sounds are played at a loud enough level and with a specific pitch or frequency from a nearby loudspeaker. (Some older readers like the author may remember the TV and radio commercials of the 1960s and 1970s asking, "Is it Memorex or Ella Fitzgerald?") When the air conditioner kicks on at night, it may cause a loose windowpane or a window blind to begin rattling. This happens because the frequency of the sounds from the loudspeaker or the air conditioner is close to that of the natural resonant frequency of the water glass or the window blind. When we get to the chapters on anatomy and physiology of the ear, we will see that this natural resonant frequency phenomenon as it relates to differences in the density/stiffness characteristics of different parts of the auditory structures can explain many normal as well as abnormal characteristics of human hearing sensitivity.

It is very important that the reader understand that whenever an object is forced to vibrate at its natural resonant frequency, the amount of vibratory energy may be increased beyond what was transferred to it by the external force (thus the breaking of water glasses and the rattling of windowpanes). Engineers who build suspension bridges have known about this phenomenon for many years. The different parts of a suspension bridge, when taken together, have a specific combined stiffness and, ergo, a natural resonant frequency. In a mild windstorm, such bridges have been known to begin vibrating to such an extent that they literally tear apart and collapse. This is because the frequency of the vibratory energy created in the surrounding air molecules by the storm is close to that of the bridge's natural resonant frequency.

Finally, before turning to a description of the anatomy and physiology of the auditory system, the author must explain how the amplitudes or "physical strength" of sounds are measured. He has been doing this, at least once a year, for the past 30+ years, and has yet to find a means of teaching this subject without inflicting some degree of pain and frustration on his students (hopefully, decreasing in magnitude over the years as the author improved his teaching skills). Sound amplitudes are measured in decibels. The scale of measurement used for decibels is a ratio scale. Very few students, or professors for that matter, have ever had any direct contact with ratio scales. Most of us are very familiar with nominal, ordinal, and interval scales of measurement. Almost everyone, however, is confused when first encountering the concept of the decibel. The reason we have to do this is that humans, and many of our nonhuman relatives, have extremely sensitive auditory systems. If our ears were any more sensitive, we would literally be able to hear air molecules crashing into each other (the so-called random Brownian movement of air molecules). The physical intensity range of sounds from those we can barely hear (threshold) to the level that is uncomfortable or possibly damaging is *huge*! Depending on which expert you believe, or how many zeros you can write before getting writer's cramp, that range may be as large as the number 10 followed by 14 zeros to 1 (i.e., 100,000,000,000,000 to 1). Audiologists find this intensity scale, although it is an interval or linear scale, to be totally unmanageable for purposes of measuring and reporting human thresholds. In many textbooks, the authors proceed to explain the concept of the decibel using very technical terms like logarithms, dynes, and micropascals, combined with equally obtuse and frustrating mathematical formulae. As with the earlier description of pure tones or sine waves, the author will again attempt to explain the concept of the decibel in nontechnical layman's terms. However, readers may want to turn to the more technical descriptions in other textbooks as a means of assisting them in understanding the decibel.

If audiologists had to deal with a 100,000,000,000,000 to 1 interval scale to measure and report the hearing sensitivity of their patients, they would probably throw up their hands and quit. Fortunately, many years ago some hearing scientist came up with an ingenious solution to this dilemma. Those readers who are mathematically oriented may have noticed that the number 10 followed by 14 zeros is the same thing as "raising 10 to the power of 14," or 10^{14}. The number 14 is actually a logarithm. The scientist then used the number 14 and developed the so-called Bel scale (named in honor of Alexander Graham Bell, the inventor of the telephone). This new Bel scale now ranged from 14 to 1.

This scale, however, did not work for very long. Anybody can tell you that a scale that has a range of only 14 points cannot possibly account for the wide expanse of sound intensities we all encounter in our daily lives. The scientist thought for a nanosecond and then came up with the idea of multiplying this intensity range by a factor of 10 and making it 140 to 1. This new scale was named the decibel scale. However, whereas the old 100,000,000,000,000 to 1 scale was an interval or linear scale, the new scale is a ratio scale. Table 1–1 illustrates how these two scales are related. Therein lies

Table 1–1. Shows how the extremely wide dynamic range of normal human hearing is transformed into a much narrower (albeit complex ratio) scale of measurement that audiologists can more easily manage for purposes of clinically describing normal hearing versus hearing loss in their patients

PHYSICAL INTENSITY (Interval scale)	BEL SCALE (Logarithm)	DECIBEL SCALE (BEL Scale × 10)
1	0	0
10	1	10
100	2	20
1000	3	30
10000	4	40
↓	↓	↓
100000000000000	14	140

the problem that has haunted students and teachers of hearing science ever since. Whereas interval scales have equal intervals between various points on the scale, ratio scales do not. Two common interval scales that the reader is very familiar with are height and weight. If someone is 3 feet tall, he is one half the height of someone who is 6 feet tall, and someone who weighs 220 pounds is twice as heavy as someone who weighs 110 pounds. However, the points on the decibel scale do not have equal intervals. As you go from the low end of 1 dB upward towards 140 dB, each successive interval gets larger and larger. A change from 10 to 20 dB represents a much smaller change of intensity than does a change from 60 to 70. If the audiologist measures one person's detection threshold, for example for 1000 Hz tones, to be 50 dB HL (which would represent an approximate 25 dB hearing loss, given that 25 dB HL is considered normal), someone who has double this loss would not have a threshold of 100 dB HL but would have a threshold of 56 dB HL.

Before ending our discussion of the decibel scale, the author needs to make a few more critical points to round out the reader's understanding of this scale. The decibel scale that audiologists and practicing SLPs use was invented to fit the range of sounds heard by normal young human listeners. It does not work well with your cat or dog. For the really high frequencies (above about 20,000 Hz), whereas you and I may be insensitive to these sounds, your best friend (a.k.a., the family cat or dog) can hear them quite well. When we get to the anatomy and physiology chapter, we will explain why this is so. As a clue, it has something to do with the natural resonant frequency of objects (in this case, your pet's and our ear structures). Cats or dogs, being smaller than humans, have ear structures that, although virtually identical to ours, are smaller and tend to be somewhat stiffer. Because of this, their ears will allow somewhat higher frequency sounds to pass (be transmitted) through the system than will ours.

In measuring the amplitudes of sounds, hearing scientists and acoustical engineers use one of two procedures. The most commonly used procedure is to measure the pressure that the vibrating air molecules produce when they push against the eardrum or the microphone diaphragm of a sound level recording instrument. Thus, the sound pressure level (or SPL for short) is what is most typically reported in scientific journals or textbooks. Many acoustical engineers, on the other hand, prefer to use an intensity level (IL for short). (The reader needs to be forewarned that most audiologists, including the author, tend to use the terms *intensity* and *amplitude* interchangeably as informal descriptors of the "strength" of sounds when, in fact, virtually 100% of the time they are actually talking about SPL levels. Physicists always distinguish between the IL and SPL modes of measurement.) When reporting sound intensities verbally or in written reports, all engineers or hearing scientists must specify which procedure (or reference) was used, whether IL or SPL. To report a dB level by itself is not accurate. They must report it as a dB IL or a dB SPL to be totally accurate. Both the IL and SPL methods use the same 140 to 1 scale, but typically the SPL "readings" are double that of the IL readings. For example, if you have a 40 dB SPL sound and want to double it, you would increase the level to 46 dB SPL. If you were using the IL system, the 40 dB IL level would become 43 dB IL. For practical purposes, students of audiology and SLPs do not need to be bothered by these differences between the IL and SPL methods of measurement.

Now, for one additional piece of information on the quirkiness of the decibel scale. The 1 on the 140 to 1 scale represents the average thresholds of healthy adult (human) listeners. The number 140, however, represents a point where the sounds are usually very uncomfortably loud or possibly damaging to the system. The audiologist may, with many healthy children, report that the threshold is 0 or even below 0, perhaps –5 or –10. These numbers do not mean that sound is absent, but that the child has hearing that is more sensitive than the young adults' that were originally tested for purposes of developing the scale.

Now, having totally confused the reader by talking about how the scientists and engineers measure and report the decibel levels of sounds, the author needs to forewarn the reader that yet another scale of threshold measure has been invented by the clinical audiologist to simplify the task of comparing the hearing sensitivity of the patient's hearing at different pure tone frequencies. This scale, which was alluded to earlier in the present text, is called the hearing level (or HL scale for short). It was invented to avoid the complication that normal young adults are more sensitive to pure tones in the middle frequency range (e.g., 1000 and 2000 Hz) than at higher (8000 Hz) or lower (125 Hz) frequencies. Today's clinical audiometers have their internal electronic circuits adjusted so that 0 dB HL, or 10 dB HL, etc., represent the same starting levels independent of differences in expected normal thresholds. Thus, a patient could have a 60 dB HL hearing threshold level at both 250 Hz and 2000 Hz, which would indicate a similar "hearing loss" of 35 dB (since audiologists usually consider 25 dB HL as "normal") in spite of the fact that the human ear is normally more sensitive to 2000 than to 250 Hz. The author will describe this practical HL scale in more detail when we get to the second part of the present text. Figure 1–4 depicts how the SPL scale used by hearing scientists is converted to the HL scale used by clinical audiologists.

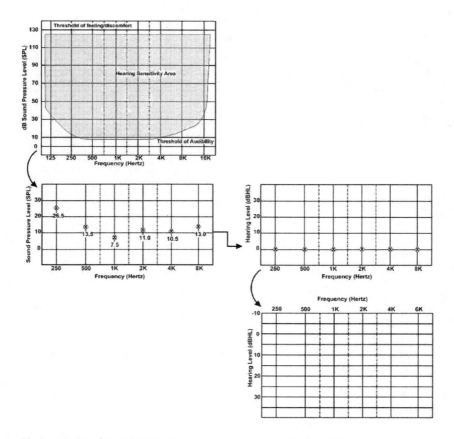

Figure 1–4. Shows how the sound pressure level (SPL) measures of human sensitivity (top left graph) used by the hearing scientist are converted to the hearing level (HL) scale developed by the audiologist (bottom right graph) for use in the hearing clinic. See the text for a description of how this conversion is accomplished.

References and Suggestions for Further Reading

There exists a large number of very excellent published sources that the reader could go to for more in-depth information related to the acoustical bases for audiology. Some sources are very simple and easy to understand, while others are extremely technical and virtually impossible for anyone but the experts to understand. The author would recommend the following sources as being useful for readers of the present text to expand their present knowledge of this area.

Durrant, J. D., & Lovrinic, J. H. (1984). *Bases of hearing science* (2nd ed., Chapters 1 to 3). Baltimore: Williams and Wilkins.

Slightly more technical but equal in depth to the Yost text. The book is older but, fortunately, acoustics has not changed much since the dinosaurs stopped pounding the ground eons ago.

Northern, J. L. (Ed.) (1996). *Hearing disorders*. Boston: Allyn and Bacon. (All editions, including third edition, Appendix, "Programmed Instruction in the Decibel," pp. 323–341)

For many years, the author has been requiring his students to look at and thoroughly work through this excellent self-teaching aid prepared many years ago by Dr. Charles Berlin.

Speaks, C. E. (1999). *Introduction to sound: Acoustics for the hearing and speech sciences* (3rd ed.). San Diego, CA: Singular.

An excellent but considerably more thorough and technical book that is entirely devoted to the science of acoustics. Even comes with an excellent CD-ROM containing outstanding examples of different acoustical/hearing phenomena.

Yost, W. A., (1994). *Fundamentals of hearing: An introduction* (3rd ed., Chapters 1 to 5). San Diego, CA: Academic Press.

A good general introduction to acoustics.

2

Functional Anatomy of the Auditory Nervous System

In this section of the text, the author will trace the functional steps or stages that occur from the point at which sound arrives at the pinna to that at which neural impulses arrive at the higher auditory neocortical regions for conscious perception of the sound. The emphasis will be on describing function first followed by brief overviews of the anatomical and physiological infrastructure that supports the different functions. Before going into a detailed description of each of the separate outer, middle, and inner ear structures of the hearing system, the reader should carefully examine Figure 2–1. This excellent drawing provides a detailed overview of the anatomy of each of these different structures along with their relationship to the other structures of the skull including the mastoid bone and brain.

Role of the Pinna in Hearing

In many nonhuman animal species, the pinna performs the very important role of collecting and focusing sounds down into the ear canal. Many species have large pinnae that can be moved in the direction of the sound source to facilitate the collection process. In

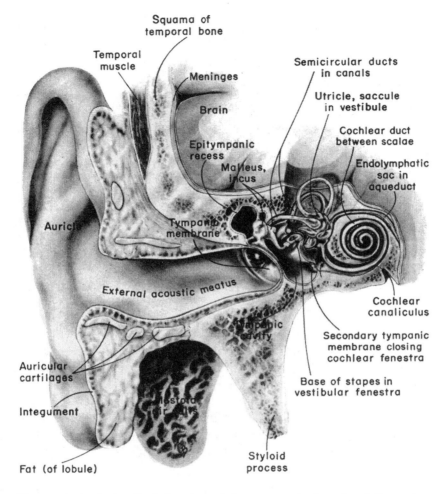

Squama of
temporal bone

Temporal
muscle

Meninges

Semicircular ducts
in canals

Brain

Utricle, saccule
in vestibule

Epitympanic
recess

Cochlear duct
between scalae

Malleus,
incus

Endolymphatic
sac in
aqueduct

Auricle

Tympanic
membrane

External acoustic meatus

Cochlear
canaliculus

Tympanic
cavity

Secondary tympanic
membrane closing
cochlear fenestra

Auricular
cartilages

Base of stapes in
vestibular fenestra

Integument

Fat (of lobule)

Styloid
process

Figure 2–1. A detailed drawing of the anatomical parts of the outer, middle, and inner ear. Modified from *Surgical Anatomy of the Temporal Bone and Ear* (p. 158) by B. J. Anson and J. A. Donaldson, Philadelphia: W. B. Saunders. Copyright 1973.

elephants it is interesting that the pinna performs a very different but important role in cooling the blood and protecting the animal from excessive heat. In man, probably the most important role is holding up eyeglasses and sunglasses or hanging small (or large) decorative ornaments (Figure 2–2). The uneven surface of the pinna

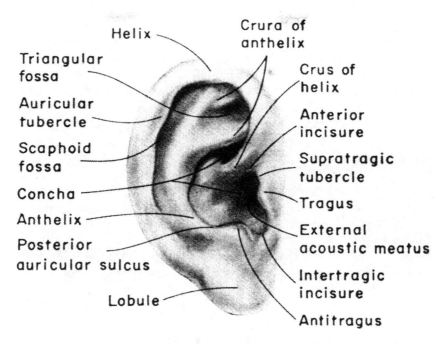

Figure 2–2. The human pinna. While this structure may assist some mammalian species in collecting and amplifying sounds, its role in man is rudimentary. The pinna does, however, provide its owner with some subtle learned cues (due to slight alterations of loudness and pitch of sounds) for locating sounds in the midline (directly in front, overhead, or directly behind the head). Reprinted from *Surgical Anatomy of the Temporal Bone and Ear* (p. 160) by B. J. Anson and J. A. Donaldson, Philadelphia: W. B. Saunders. Copyright 1973.

(the hills and valleys or convolutions) provides a very primitive means of collecting some sounds, and some people have inherited the vestigial ability to move their ears, although this talent probably causes more chuckles than anything else.

Complex sounds arriving at the pinna contain many pure tones (sine waves) of changing frequency and intensity. Low-frequency sounds have larger distances between the regions of rarefaction and condensation than do higher frequencies. This is referred to as the wavelength of the individual pure tone component. This wavelength factor interacts with the differing distances between the peaks and valleys of convolutions of the pinna to allow some sounds to be better channeled (due to reflection) down into the ear canal than other sounds. Those frequencies that are channeled down to the entrance of the ear canal increase slightly in amplitude while other frequencies that tend to be reflected away from the pinna may lose some intensity when arriving at the ear canal. It has been estimated that the maximum amount of sound amplification resulting from this process in man is exceedingly small, probably amounting to no more than 2 or 3 dB, and it is limited to only certain frequencies, typically 2000 to 7000 Hz (Pickles, 1988). However, this small channeling or focusing process does slightly change the quality of the complex sound, and can be used to assist in localization of sounds in space. Sounds coming from the front of the head are perceived as qualitatively different from sounds originating directly overhead or from behind the head. The reader can demonstrate the role of the pinna by listening to the same sounds coming from different directions while alternately cupping a hand behind the pinna.

Role of the External Ear Canal

The anatomical structures that compose the functional organ of hearing in man are housed inside the temporal bone portion of the skull (Figure 2–3A). The external canal, which begins at the concha and ends at the tympanic membrane (Figure 2–3B), is curved to give the eardrum some small amount of protection from objects coming in directly from the outside. The external two thirds of the canal consists of a skin layer overlying cartilage, while the internal one third consists of skin overlying bone (the skull). As long as the ear canal remains relatively unoccluded, sound waves are not impeded on the way to the eardrum. If excessive cerumen (earwax) is present, some blockage of the canal will occur resulting in some small amount of hearing loss. If the canal wall is completely collapsed on itself, or the patient has a form of ear canal atresia (absence of the canal), considerably more hearing loss will result.

Because of the phenomenon of natural resonant frequency, certain frequency components of any complex (multiple frequency mix of sine waves, such as speech) sound will be slightly amplified or enhanced by the time they arrive at the tympanic membrane. The concha (entrance to canal) and various portions of the ear canal

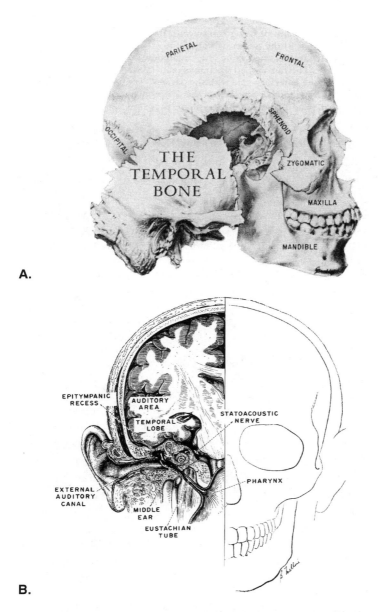

A.

B.

Figure 2–3. Depicts the anatomical relationship between the outer, middle, and inner ear and temporal bone and skull. (**A**) Shows the location of the temporal bone portion of the skull that houses the middle ear and inner ear structures. From *The Surgical Anatomy of the Temporal Bone and Ear* (p. xvii), by B. J. Anson and J. A. Donaldson, Philadelphia: W. B. Saunders. Copyright 1973. (**B**) Depicts the parts of the ear relative to the other parts of the face and skull. Courtesy of Abbott Laboratories.

each have, because of differences in density/stiffness, different resonant frequency properties. Although individual variability exists from one person's ear to another, the combined resonant frequency properties of the entire canal produce as much as a 10 to 15 dB SPL passive amplification in sound energy for the frequency range from close to 2000 to 5000 Hz (Shaw, 1974; Pickles, 1988). It is interesting that the range of frequencies that gets boosted lies right in the middle of the critical frequency range for speech sounds. This "passive amplification" phenomenon is due to the fact that whenever the natural resonant frequency of the vibrating air molecules matches the natural resonant frequency of individual parts of the ear canal, additional energy will be created and exit the structures. Thus, the ear contains its own built-in "hearing aid," at least for the speech frequencies. Figure 2–4 depicts how the different natural resonant properties of the human ear canal provide amplification for sounds in the normal speech frequency range.

Role of the Middle Ear System

The middle ear system, which is housed in the temporal bone region of the skull (see Figure 2–3A), consists of an enclosed space that, except for a tube (known as the eustachian tube) that connects this space to the inside of the back part of the mouth (known technically as the nasopharynx, located close to the adenoids and tonsils), would be closed off from the outside world. Figure 2–5 provides two illustrative views of the canal and makeup of the middle ear space. Most of the time, the eustachian tube stays open or can be easily opened to allow equalization of air pressure between the middle ear space and the outside world. Because of the proximity of this tube to the adenoids and tonsils, throat infections (or allergies) can cause these structures to swell and keep the eustachian tube closed. This can trigger a chain of pathological events (middle ear infections, accumulation of fluid in the middle ear space, ruptured eardrums, etc.) that can impair the patient's hearing sensitivity.

The lateral wall of the middle ear space (adjacent to the ear canal) consists of the relatively large tympanic membrane (TM). The TM consists of an outer skin layer that is continuous with the skin layer of the external ear canal and an inner skin layer that is continuous with the mucous membrane ("wet skin") layer of the middle ear space.

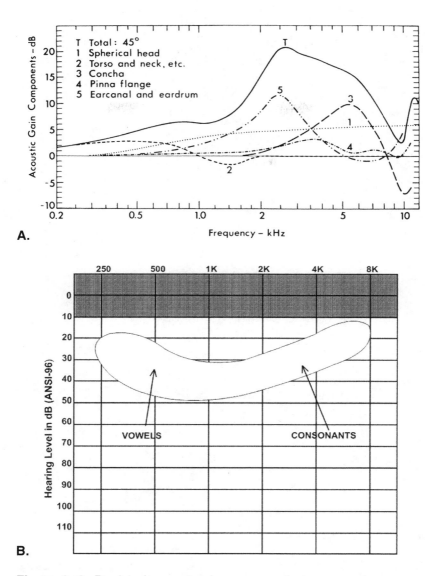

Figure 2–4. Depicts how natural resonance frequency enhances our hearing of sounds in the normal speech range. (**A**) Shows how the different parts of the ear from the pinna to the tympanic membrane (including, to a smaller degree, the head plus torso and neck) act to passively amplify (via natural resonance) incoming sounds. Reprinted with permission from the "External Ear" by E. A. G. Shaw, in W. D. Keidel and W. D. Neff, Eds., *Handbook of Sensory Physiology* (p. 468), Berlin: Springer-Verlag. Copyright 1974. (**B**) Shows that the frequencies amplified the most cover the range of the basic low-frequency vowel and higher frequency consonant sounds of human speech.

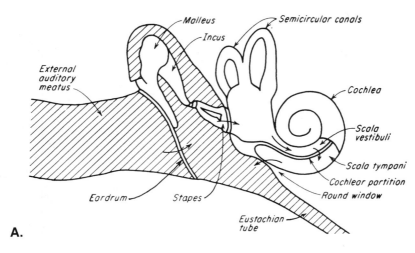

A.

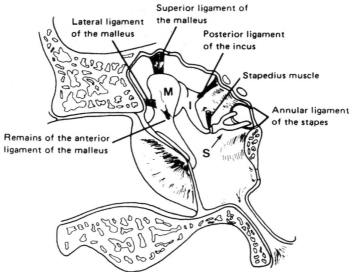

B.

Figure 2–5. Two different views of the relative locations of the outer, middle, and inner ear structures. (**A**) Reproduced with permission from *Experiments in Hearing* (p. 11) by G. Von Bekesy, New York: McGraw-Hill. Copyright 1960. (**B**) Illustrates the relative locations of the different structures of the middle ear including the different ligaments that are suspended from the walls and ceiling of the middle ear space to hold the three ossicles in place. Also shown is the stapedius muscle that attaches to the head of the stapes. Reprinted with permission from *Speech and Hearing Sciences: Anatomy and Physiology* (3rd ed., Fig. 6–57, p. 448), by W. Zemlin, Englewood Cliffs, NJ: Prentice-Hall. Copyright 1988.

In between the two skin layers can be found a series of both radial and circular cartilaginous fibers that gives the TM some toughness and resistance to tearing. A chain of three separate small bones, the malleus, incus, and stapes, is positioned between the larger TM and a much smaller membrane (known as the oval window). The oval window separates the normally air filled middle ear space from the fluid filled inner ear or cochlea. The larger of the three bones, the malleus, is attached to the approximate middle of the TM. A large portion of the TM (approximately 55 of its total of 85 square centimeters) is tightly attached to the malleus (analogous to a drum head) so that the malleus and approximately two thirds of the TM vibrate as one unit. The remaining one third of the surface of the TM is not tightly attached to the malleus, and when the malleus moves, this loose part of the TM "goes along for the ride." The total area of the TM that vibrates is 14 times larger than the total area of the oval window membrane.

The three ear bones (sometimes referred to as the *hammer, anvil,* and *stirrup* because of the similarity of their shapes to these common tools) are hinged with each other by flexible joints (not unlike an elbow or knee joint) so that each can, to some degree, move independently of the other two. The three ossicles are supported by a series of ligaments (Figure 2–5B) that are attached to the walls and ceiling of the middle ear space. This makes the ossicular chain structurally very similar to a suspension bridge. Because of this, they are very vulnerable to trauma or disease (for example, accumulation of middle ear fluid). Thus, the ossicles are suspended by ligaments, hinged and able to move independently of each other, and the malleus is the largest of the three, and the stapes is the smallest and lightest of the three. Figure 2–6 contrasts the size of the ossicles to that of a U.S. penny.

Prior to the initiation of biochemical related nerve impulses in the inner ear, sounds undergo two physical transformations. The first is an air-to-vibratory transformation in which some physical disturbance causes air molecules to switch from their normal random vibratory pattern (Brownian movement) to a systematic movement of regions of alternating condensation (higher air pressure, more molecules per unit volume) and rarefaction (lower air pressure, fewer molecules per unit volume). The second is a vibratory-to-mechanical transformation, which occurs when the air molecules push against the eardrum to begin the to and fro mechanical pushing

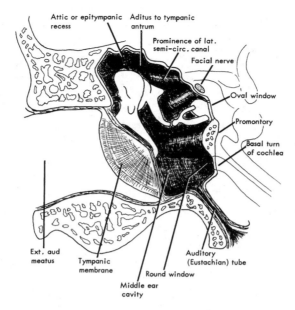

A.

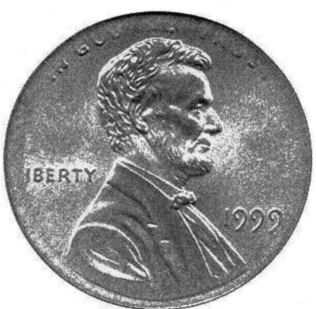

B.

Figure 2–6. (**A**) Schematic drawing of the middle ear. Reproduced with permission from *Speech and Hearing Sciences: Anatomy and Physiology* (3rd ed., Fig. 6–44, p. 439), by W. Zemlin, Englewood Cliffs, NJ: Prentice-Hall. Copyright 1988. (**B**) Illustrates the size of the middle ear structures in relation to the size of a U.S. penny.

of the ossicles and, in particular, the stapes against the oval window membrane. However, the fact that the inner ear is filled with fluid means that sounds that begin as vibrating air molecules must eventually become vibrating fluid molecules in order to allow the next step in the chain of events related to stimulating nerve impulses. Air is a lower density and much less stiff medium than is fluid. The transmission of energy from one medium to another medium that has a different density and, ergo, a different natural resonant frequency, requires more energy. This is technically termed an impedance mismatch between the two mediums. Thus, if we tried to transmit the energy of vibrating air molecules directly into a fluid medium, only about 1% of the energy would be transferred. An incredible 99% would be reflected away from the fluid and lost (Figure 2–7). In terms of the decibel scale, this would translate into a 40 dB HL hearing loss (if you were listening for the airborne sounds with your head under water). The reader needs to understand that, whenever there is an impedance mismatch between two adjacent mediums (such as air and water), the loss of energy is the same whether the vibrations are traveling from the stiffer to the less stiff medium, or vice versa. Thus, if a person who is underwater shouts to his friend who is sitting on the river bank, only 1% of the

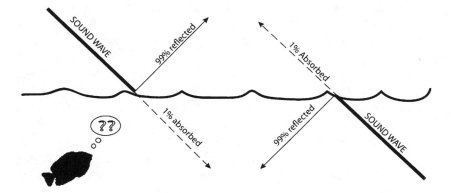

Figure 2–7. Illustrates the physical impedance mismatch between air and water. Note that the transfer of vibratory energy from a less dense medium (air) to a denser medium is a "two-way street." The same amount of impedance occurs whether energy is moving from a less to a denser medium or from a denser medium (water) to less dense air.

sound would get to the friend (perhaps the moral of this story is that drowning persons should only shout for help when their heads are above water and hold their breaths when below water).

The functional role of the middle ear system is to overcome the impedance mismatch between air and fluid. Without the middle ear system, people would not be deaf but would be walking around with a substantial 40 dB HL hearing loss. Mother Nature has provided three separate mechanisms in the middle ear to assist in overcoming this mismatch problem. Figure 2–8 shows each of these three mechanisms. The first and most important mechanism is the areal ratio difference between the tympanic membrane and the oval window membrane (Figure 2–8A). The vibrating area of the TM is 14 times larger than that of the oval window. When the airborne sounds arrive at the TM the energy is spread over a relatively large area. When this energy is transferred to the stapes, it is focused onto an area that is 14 times smaller. The same amount of energy spread over a large area (eardrum) becomes magnified when spread over a smaller area (oval window). This is why focusing sunlight with a magnifying glass will start a fire, and why it is easy to drive the small point of a nail into wood when hitting the larger head of the nail with a hammer. This areal ratio effect overcomes approximately 23 dB of the total hearing loss due to the air-fluid impedance mismatch.

The second mechanism (Figure 2–8B) for overcoming the impedance mismatch relates to the fact that, of the three ossicles, the malleus is the longest. This provides a small fulcrum advantage, not unlike that seen with a mechanical crowbar or the schoolyard teeter totter. With the teeter totter, a less heavy child can lift a heavier child if the smaller child is sitting further away than the heavier child from the point on the board that acts as the fulcrum or pivot point. This fulcrum advantage of the ossicular chain provides an approximate 1.3 to 1 advantage, which acts to amplify the sounds by another 4–5 dB.

The third mechanism (Figure 2–8C) for overcoming the normal air-to-fluid impedance mismatch problem is somewhat more difficult to explain and understand. In earlier discussions, we mentioned that approximately one third of the total area of the TM is not tightly attached to the malleus, thus giving the TM a slightly conical shape. Therefore, when the tightly stretched areas of the eardrum and the malleus move together as a unit, this smaller area of the TM tends to move somewhat independently and may initially lag behind and then suddenly catch up. This produces a buckling action of the TM.

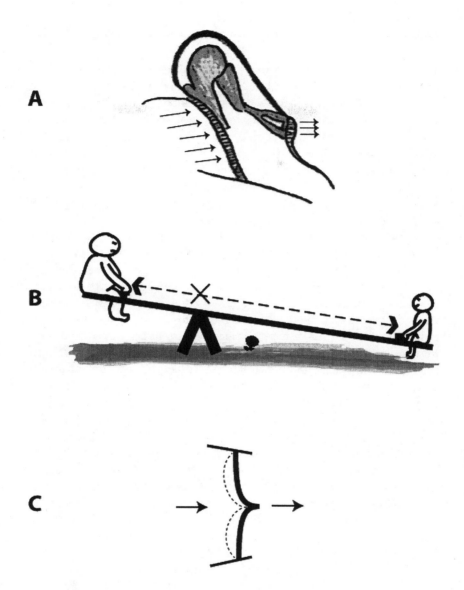

Figure 2–8. Three middle ear mechanisms that assist in overcoming the normal impedance mismatch between air and water. (**A**) The total vibratory area of the tympanic membrane is 14 times larger than the area of the oval window membrane, which allows the pressure at the oval window to be magnified by a factor of 14. (**B**) The fulcrum advantage (analogous to a crowbar) provided by the differences in length and action of the three ossicular bones. (**C**) The buckling effect provided by the separate movement of areas of the TM that are more or less tightly attached to the malleus.

This is why the action of a bullwhip produces a sudden explosion of energy similar to a gunshot. It is also why, in the shower room, when your friend flicks a towel at your derriere, it may really hurt. The whiplike movement of the loose unstretched areas of the TM provides an approximate 4 to 1 boost to the total sound energy, yielding an additional 12 dB amplification. Thus, the separate intensity boost provided by all three of the described air-fluid impedance mismatch mechanisms, when added up (23 + 5 + 12 dB), comes amazingly close to the 40 dB loss that would have been produced by the air-fluid impedance mismatch.

The author needs to emphasize that the exact magnitudes of impedance matching (23, 5, and 12 dB) presented in the preceding paragraph are not universally agreed upon by all experts in the field. Your author was a hearing scientist for many years prior to becoming a clinical audiologist. Much of his knowledge of middle ear anatomy/ physiology was derived from earlier studies with animals and, in particular, the cat. While most experts agree that the three impedance matching mechanisms listed above are probably shared by both animals (cats) and humans, the exact amount of the impedance matching associated with each mechanism probably differs, not only from one person to another, but also from one animal species to another (Pickles, 1988; Yost, 1994; Harris, 1986; Durrant & Lovrinic, 1981). The important point to understand, however, is that the middle ear system is designed to overcome some if not most of the loss of hearing that normally would occur if air conducted sound had to be directly transferred to the fluid filled inner ear space. As indicated earlier, the passive amplification features (due to resonance) of the pinna, concha, and ear canal also assist in this impedance matching task.

Role of the Inner Ear

Unlike the ear canal and the middle ear space, which is normally filled with air, the inner ear is completely filled with fluid. This fluid is chemically very similar to seawater (and to the fluid that surrounds the brain, known as cerebrospinal fluid) and is termed *perilymph*. The inner ear consists of two series of fluid-filled systems, one of which controls our balance functions (known as the vestibular system), and the other (the cochlea) controls our hearing function (Figure 2–9). The vestibular system and the cochlea are continuous

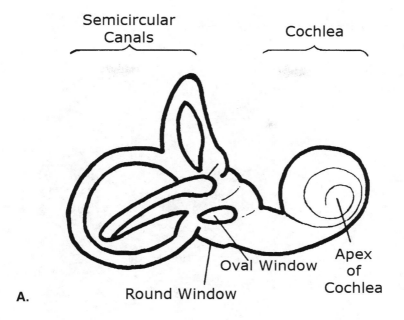

Semicircular
Canals

Cochlea

Oval Window

Round Window

Apex
of
Cochlea

A.

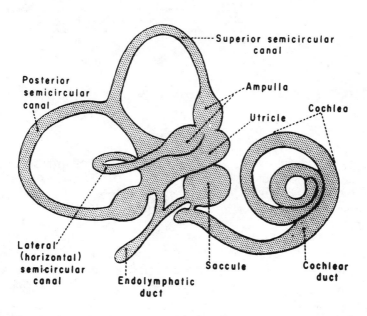

Superior semicircular
canal

Posterior
semicircular
canal

Ampulla

Utricle

Cochlea

Lateral
(horizontal)
semicircular
canal

Saccule

Cochlear
duct

Endolymphatic
duct

B.

Figure 2–9. (**A**) Depicts the gross anatomical features of the bony labyrinth. (**B**) Shows the membranous labyrinth, which is housed inside the bony labyrinth. Reproduced with permission from *Bases of Hearing Science* (p. 98), by J. D. Durrant and J. H. Lovrinic, Baltimore: Williams & Wilkins. Copyright 1977. *continues*

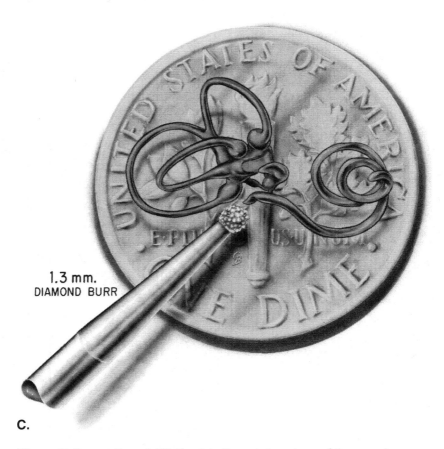

1.3 mm.
DIAMOND BURR

C.

Figure 2–9. *continued* (**C**) Depicts the relative sizes of the membranous labyrinth and a U.S. dime. Reproduced from *The Surgical Anatomy of the Temporal Bone and Ear* (p. 98), by B. J. Anson and J. A. Donaldson, Philadelphia: W. B. Saunders. Copyright 1973.

with each other and share the same fluid (perilymph), which at times can spell big troubles for patients if infections or disease processes in one system move to the other system. With some inner ear diseases, such as Ménière's disease, patients exhibit both hearing and dizziness problems. In the remainder of this text, our discussions will be focused exclusively on the cochlea and how it works (or malfunctions).

The cochlea can be thought of as a long, fluid-filled, cavelike structure (or cavern) that is carved out of the surrounding temporal bone. This cavern is referred to as the bony labyrinth, ergo, the term *cavelike* (Figure 2–9A). In order to conserve space, the cochlea is coiled up in a tight spiral configuration, which makes it resemble a snail. Throughout almost all of its length, this bony labyrinth contains a somewhat flexible tubelike structure that stretches from one side of the bony labyrinth to the other. This structure is called the membranous labyrinth (Figure 2–9B). When we reach the far end of the bony labyrinth, or the part known as the apex, we find that the membranous labyrinth does not extend all the way to the end. The apex contains a small gap, called the helicotrema. Thus, the perilymph in the bony labyrinth, both that in the chamber above (referred to as the scala vestibuli) and below (the scala tympani) the membranous labyrinth (which is also commonly known as the scala media), are continuous with each other. Because the inner ear is comprised of three separate chambers (scalae) which are coiled like a snail in a complex fashion, many new students get confused and cannot picture this relationship in their minds. A careful review of Figure 2–10 and Figure 2–11, in the sequence presented, hopefully will help to clarify this difficult anatomical relationship.

When the stapes of the middle ear pushes in and out on the flexible oval window, the fluid in the inner ear becomes alternately more and less compressed than normal (analogous to the condensation and rarefaction events related to the sound-induced vibration of air molecules). When the oval window moves inward and compresses the inner ear fluid, something has to give, so to speak. The increased pressure must be relieved somehow. In addition to the oval window, on the medial wall of the middle ear, and located slightly below the oval window, there exists a second small window covered by a flexible membrane. This window is referred to as the round window. Whereas the oval window connects with the chamber (the scala vestibuli) located above the stretched membranous labyrinth (i.e., scalae media), the round window connects with the lower chamber (scala tympani). When the oval window is pushed inward by the stapes, the resulting increased fluid pressure is relieved by a simultaneous outward movement of the round window membrane (Figure 2–12). Thus, sound that begins as vibrating air molecules (and regions of condensation or rarefaction, i.e., increased or decreased air pressure) eventually becomes alternating increases and decreases in the inner ear fluid pressure. With higher frequency sounds, the air vibrates more quickly and the regions of rarefaction

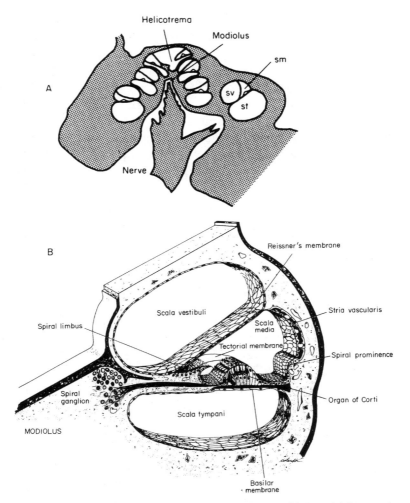

Figure 2–10. In order to conserve space, the cochlea, which consists of a long, tunnel-like structure (bony labyrinth that houses the smaller membranous labyrinth), is coiled on itself and closely resembles a snail. A horizontal cross section taken through the middle of the coiled cochlea will resemble a treelike structure. The exiting 8th cranial (or vestibular-auditory) nerve will look like the trunk of the tree, and the series of holes in the mastoid bone (the bony labyrinth) will be broad at the base of the tree and come to a peak at the location of the helicotrema. (**A**) Depicts the tree analogy of this cross section through the cochlea. Abbreviations: sv, scala vestibuli; sm, scala media; st, scala tympani. (**B**) Shows a magnified view of one of the holes in the mastoid bone that shows the complex anatomical nature of the contents of the bony and membranous labyrinths. Both A and B are reproduced with permission from *A Textbook of Histology* (fig 35.11), by D. W. Fawcett, London: Arnold Publishers. Copyright 1986.

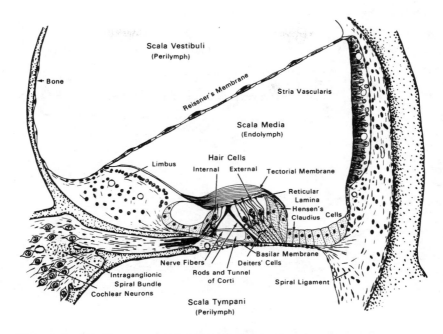

Figure 2–11. Shows a detailed schematic drawing of the anatomical structures of the basilar membrane and organ of Corti. Reproduced with permission from "Acoustic Trauma in the Guinea Pig," by H. Davis et al., 1953, *Journal of the Acoustical Society of America, 25*, p. 1180. Copyright 1953.

and condensation are closer together. This causes the stapes to be shoved in and out of the oval window at a faster rate. The different rates of stapes movement are the mechanical essence of differences in sound frequency. Now, how does the inner ear go about responding to these stapedial rate changes to transform this energy into nerve impulses that can allow your brain to know whether you are listening to someone singing bass, baritone, or soprano?

In the last paragraph, we said that the cochlea (which is coiled) contains a third enclosed membranous labyrinth that separates the bony labyrinth into an upper (scala vestibuli) and lower chamber (scala tympani), both filled with the same perilymph because the two chambers are connected by a small opening (helicotrema) at the apical end. The membranous labyrinth or scala media is a very complex structure that contains the critical anatomical and physiological

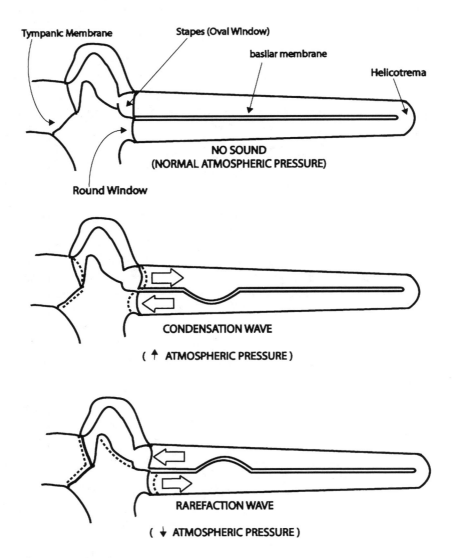

Figure 2–12. Shows how the repetitive inward and outward movement of the stapes and oval window in response to incoming sound waves produces vibratory motions of the basilar membrane (BM). In response to the condensation (increased air pressure) portion of the incoming sound wave, the stapes moves inward to produce a downward motion of the BM. In response to the rarefaction portion of the wave (decreased air pressure), the BM moves upward.

infrastructure that allows sound-induced nerve impulses to be generated and transmitted to the brain. The lower part of the scala media that stretches across the middle of the bony labyrinth is known as the basilar membrane (BM) (see Figure 2–11). At the basal end of the cochlea, the BM is narrower and more tightly stretched. At the apical end the BM is wider and less tightly stretched. As you travel through the membranous labyrinth from the basal end (the part closest to the middle ear space and separated from the middle ear space by the oval and round windows), this membrane gradually increases in width by a factor of 10 and decreases its stiffness by a factor of 100 (Figure 2–13). Because of the phenomenon of natural resonant frequency, the BM has a unique tonotopic organization. Depending on the natural resonant frequency of any particular segment of the BM, different frequency sounds (i.e., different rates of inward and outward movement of the stapes) can more easily make the BM vibrate than other frequencies. Because of this gradient in stiffness along the length of the BM, the basal end will vibrate more easily to high frequency sounds and the apical end will vibrate more easily to low frequency sounds (Figure 2–14). This tonotopic phenomenon related to the pattern of basilar membrane vibration is referred to as the *traveling wave theory of hearing.*

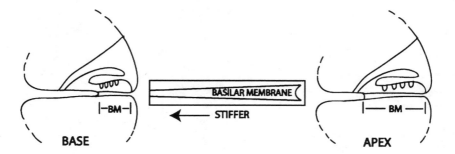

Figure 2–13. Between the base (location of stapes and oval window) and apex (helicotrema), the basilar membrane (cochlear partition) gradually decreases in stiffness by a factor of 100 and increases in width by a factor of 10.

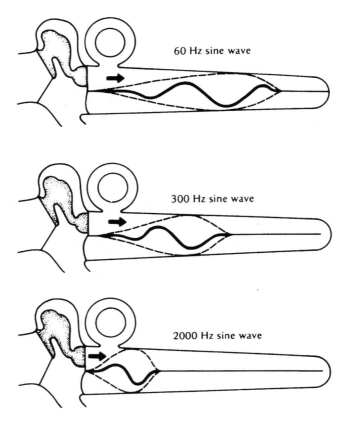

Figure 2–14. The peak of the traveling wave produced on the basilar membrane occurs closer to the base with increases in sound frequency, and closer to the apex in response to lower frequency sounds. Reproduced with permission from *Speech and Hearing Sciences: Anatomy and Physiology* (3rd ed., Fig. 6–101, p. 479), by W. Zemlin, Englewood Cliffs, NJ: Prentice-Hall. Copyright 1988.

Sitting on top of the BM, there exists a very complex structure know as the organ of Corti (Figure 2–15A; also see Figure 2–11). This structure is continuous throughout the entire length of the BM from base to apex. There is a small membrane (Reissner's membrane, see Figure 2–11) that is situated above the organ of Corti that acts to completely separate this complex structure (i.e., the scala media) from the scala vestibuli and scala tympani. Reissner's mem-

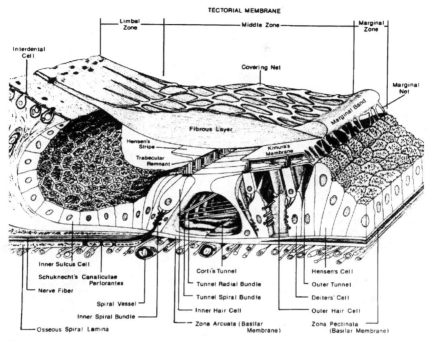

A.

Figure 2–15. (A) Shows how all structures of the organ of Corti are continuous from the base to the apex. A single row of inner hair cells and three or four rows of outer hair cells are lined up underneath the overhanging tectorial membrane along the entire length of the basilar membrane. Reproduced with permission from "Cochlear Anatomy Related to Cochlear Micromechanics: A review," by D. J. Lim, 1980, *Journal of the Acoustical Society of America, 67*, pp. 1686–1695. Copyright 1980. *continues*

brane seals off the organ of Corti from the surrounding perilymph-filled chambers. The membranous labyrinth or scala media is filled with a special fluid, known as endolymph, which has a different chemical composition from the perilymph in the other two chambers. The endolymph is important in allowing nerve impulses to be generated. Any tear to Reissner's membrane that might allow the perilymph and endolymph to mix would have dire consequences for the patient's hearing.

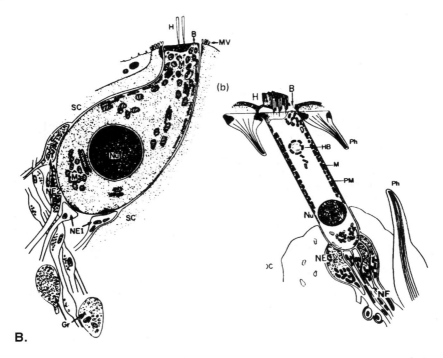

B.

Figure 2–15. *continued* (**B**) Shows schematics of the structure of the inner (*left drawing*) and outer (*right drawing*) hair cells. Reproduced with permission from *Physiological Bases of Medical Practice*, J. R. Brodbeck (Ed.), Baltimore: Williams & Wilkins. Copyright 1973.

The organ of Corti contains the specialized hair cells that are the source of the neural impulses that travel to the higher centers of the brain to announce the arrival of sounds. There are two types of hair cells known as the inner and outer hair cells (Figure 2–15B). The average human cochlea contains approximately 20,000 outer hair cells and 3500 inner hair cells. The outer hair cells are arranged in three or four adjacent rows that run the entire length of the cochlea from base to apex. The inner hair cells consist of a single row that runs the entire length of the cochlea. The positions of the inner and outer hair cells are maintained on the organ of Corti by a collection of special supporting cells. The function of the supporting cells is to make sure both types of hair cells stay upright. On the top of both type of cells, there are small hairlike structures (stereocilia) that are stiff and stick straight up. Directly above the inner and outer hair cells is a special structure known as the tectorial membrane. This membrane, which is soft and approximately the consistency of Jello, also runs the entire length of the cochlea. It overhangs and is positioned directly above the hair cell stereocilia, some of which are actually attached to the underside of this structure. Now, how do the hair cells get stimulated and generate nerve impulses?

When the stapes moves inward, it causes a temporary increased fluid pressure in the top scala vestibuli chamber. This causes the entire scala media and all its contents to be pushed downward (Figure 2–16). When the stapes moves outward, the pressure in the bottom chamber (scala tympani) temporarily becomes greater than that in the top chamber and the scala media is pushed upward. Thus, inward and outward movements of the stapes cause alternating downward and upward movement of the scala media. It is important to note that the "hinge point" of the tectorial membrane is different from that of the BM, which houses the organ of Corti and the hair cells. Because of this, when the entire scala media begins to be pushed up and down by the perilymph pressure changes, a shearing action occurs between the tectorial membrane and the underlying stereocilia of the hair cells, which causes the stereocilia to be bent alternately medially and laterally. The reader can demonstrate this shearing action by placing hands together, palms together (in a prayer mode), but with the two hands out of alignment so that the fingers of one hand stick our more and the palm of the other hand sits further back. Now, begin flexing your wrists back and forth. If you have done this correctly, you will notice that, as you move your wrists, your fingers will rub against each other. This is the same shearing action that occurs in the inner ear. The bending of the stereocilia of the hair cells causes complex biochemical changes in the inner hair cell that act to trigger a single action potential. It is only when the stereocilia of the inner hair cells are moving in the medial direction or the scala media is moving upward that the action potential is triggered. Thus, with each complete cycle of stapes movement, inward and outward, the inner hair cell elicits one action potential. If the stapes moves in and out at a rate of, for example, 250 Hz (or cps), the hair cell will respond by eliciting 250 action potentials per second. Lower frequency sounds will trigger more activity in the hair cells located close to the apical part of the BM, and higher frequency sounds will trigger more

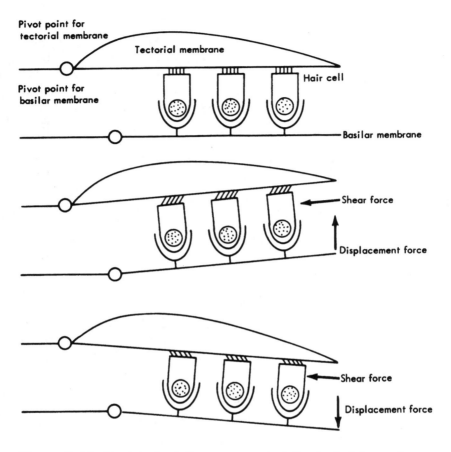

Figure 2–16. Depicts how the movement of the tectorial membrane produces a shearing action that causes a bending of the stereocilia on top of the hair cells. Reproduced with permission from *Speech and Hearing Science: Anatomy and Physiology* (3rd ed., Fig. 6–111, p. 484), by W. R. Zemlin, Englewood Cliffs, NJ: Prentice-Hall. Copyright 1988.

activity in the basal regions of the BM. Nerve fibers that are connected to the hair cells at different locations on the BM exit the inner ear and form a bundle of nerves known as the 8th cranial nerve, which then enters the brainstem and begins its journey to the higher neural centers of the brain.

For many years, scientists were puzzled by why there appeared to be two different kinds of hair cells in the inner ear. The two types of cells have different shapes (the inner hair cells shaped like a wine glass, and the outer hair cells like a rod or piston), there are 20,000 outer and only 3500 inner cells, and the two types even have a different pattern of connection with the higher parts of the brain. Inner hair cells exhibit more of a one-to-one connection, in which nerves exiting the cochlea and going to the brain are only connected to limited regions of the BM. This type of topographic arrangement is what we would intuitively expect if the individual fibers were conveying frequency-specific information. The neural inflow and outflow from the outer hair cells, in contrast, seems to be more random. Neurons coming from the brain branch extensively and tend to be connected to wide regions of the BM in a distinctly nontopographic manner. Thus, there is considerable evidence that the functional roles of the inner and outer hair cells are very different.

For years, hundreds of hearing scientists in laboratories all over the world were engaged in research to determine what kinds of functional differences existed between the inner and outer hair cells. Since both types of cells were located in the same part of the cochlea and both apparently had neural connections with higher neural centers, the overriding assumption was that both types of cells were engaged in sensory functions. Scientists believed that the two types of cells were involved in sending different kinds of sensory information to the brain. The author could write another entire book on this very interesting saga in the history of hearing science. It is an extremely fascinating story that rivals that of the discovery of the double helix makeup of the DNA molecule (Watson, 1968). However, whereas the genetics researchers were on a correct path, our hearing science friends eventually found out they had been on a totally dead end path that went nowhere.

To make a long story short, the outcome of this massive attack on the nature of inner versus outer hair cells resulted in the finding that only the inner hair cells were involved in sensory hearing function. The outer cells turned out to have an active motor function related to increasing the dynamic range of hearing. It is the outer hair cells that allow us to have such an incredibly wide range of sensitivity related to sound intensity. The student can blame the outer hair cells for the need to invent that horrible decibel amplitude scale. When sounds are relatively loud, at or above approximately 50 dB HL, the amount of vibration of the scala media and all its contents (e.g., BM, hair cells, overhanging tectorial membrane) is sufficient to cause the stereocilia on the inner hair cells to be bent and for the inner hair cells to trigger neural action potentials. When sound intensities drop below about 50 dB HL and the sounds become harder to hear, the inner hair cells cease to function because the shearing action of the tectorial membrane is no longer sufficient to bend the stereocilia. At this point the outer hair cells kick in to increase the amount of vibration of the tectorial membrane so that the stereocilia of the inner hair cells can continue to be bent and action potentials elicited. The stereocilia of the outer hair cells are imbedded in the underside of the tectorial membrane, and the outer hair cell is shaped like a rod or piston (for a good reason). When sounds get too soft to allow the inner hair cells to work, the outer hair cells begin shoving on the tectorial membrane to increase its movement, which in turn allows the inner hair cells to continue doing their thing.

Although the scientific evidence now seems well established that outer hair cells provide a unique motor function that allows us to hear a much wider range of sound intensities, scientists are only just beginning to understand the whys and hows of this very important and complex phenomenon. However, when the motor role of the outer hair cells was discovered, it suddenly unleashed explanations for a large number of curious hearing phenomena that had long puzzled audiologists and scientists alike. Taking certain *ototoxic* drugs plus long-term exposure to loud sounds are both known to produce hearing loss. The hearing loss does not involve generalized deafness for all sounds, but only for what would normally be the softer or less intense sounds. Persons with this form of hearing loss, which is frequently labeled a *recruiting hearing loss*, find that they can still hear the louder sounds that are above approximately 50 dB HL or so in intensity, but they cannot hear the softer sounds. The reason for this is that ototoxic drugs and over-exposure to noise both selectively destroy the outer hair cells but leave the inner hair cells intact. Thus, the loss of the outer hair cells removes our normal sensitivity to the lower parts of our normally very wide dynamic range of hearing. Persons who have their outer hair cells destroyed find that the normally wide range between very soft and very loud sounds is drastically reduced and even small changes in the intensity of sounds will appear exaggerated and uncomfortable (thus the term *recruitment*).

The discovery of the motor role of the outer hair cells also opened the door for the development of a new diagnostic clinical tool for the audiologist. When the outer hair cells kick in to push against the overhanging tectorial membrane, they produce vibrations in the inner ear fluids, and these vibrations will move out through the oval window, through the ossicular chain, and cause the eardrum to disturb the air molecules in the external canal. This normal function of the outer hair cells thus produces it own unique sounds that can be picked up by a very sensitive microphone placed next to the TM in the ear canal. These so-called *Kemp echoes*, named after David Kemp who first discovered them (Kemp, 1978), can be recorded and analyzed to determine if they are present and have normal features or characteristics. Audiologists refer to this new clinical tool as measurement of otoacoustic emissions. Much more will be said about this important clinical procedure when, in Part II of this book, we turn to describing what audiologists do to justify their salaries.

Role of the Higher Central Auditory Pathways

It is a truism that hearing scientists know a great deal more about the functions of the lower peripheral (outer, middle, and inner ear or cochlea) portions of the auditory nervous system than they do about the higher centers. Once the inner hair cells begin firing, and nerve impulses begin traveling upstream to the brainstem and the various higher centers of the nervous system, our level of understanding plummets. However, in addition to testing for lower level impairments in the conductive and sensory aspects of basic hearing, the audiologist may also test for disturbances in the higher level conscious or perceptual aspects of hearing. In the present text, the author will not go into a detailed description of the anatomy and physiology of the central auditory pathways, except to indicate that the system involves a multitude of different centers and neural pathways, beginning in the brainstem and ending in the neocortex, where we believe various aspects of the complex analyses and conscious perception of sounds occur. Figure 2–17 shows the various pathways and neural centers of the central portion of the auditory system. Given our present level of understanding of the functions

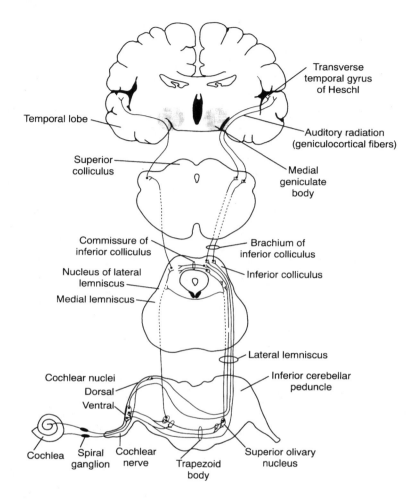

Figure 2–17. Schematic representation of the various subcortical and cortical neural centers, plus interconnecting neural pathways, that provide a series of stages for the complex sensory processing of incoming sounds at the cochlea. Reproduced with permission from *Neuroscience for the Study of Communicative Disorders* (p. 172), by S. C. Bhatnagar and O. J. Andy, Baltimore: Williams & Wilkins. Copyright 1995.

of each of the different higher neural centers, the audiologist cannot do much better than administer a battery of tests (a collection of different tests) that he or she believes can collectively distinguish peripheral from central dysfunction. The tests can assist us in determining whether the hearing problems of the patient are due to peripheral level dysfunctions related to the conduction of sounds from the outside world through the outer and middle ear system, or to inner ear sensory problems (e.g., loss of inner or outer hair cells), or, alternately, to central level problems related to the interpretation and understanding of the sounds.

References and Suggestions for Further Reading

The present textbook has been written as a very general introduction to a very complex subject matter (or collection of topics). A virtual mountain of information and facts has been presented in the preceding pages related to the functional anatomy and physiology of the auditory nervous system. The author has attempted, whenever citing specific facts (e.g., numbers of inner and outer hair cells, the amount of acoustic gain provided by the resonance properties of the ear canal, the degree of air-to-fluid impedance matching provided by the three middle ear transformation systems) to use numbers or specific information that appears to be common knowledge or at least agreed upon by the majority of experts in the field. Please do not think that the author is engaging in any form of intended plagiarism by not always citing specific references. When the information is relatively new to the profession, or somewhat controversial, the author has included specific references. However, the author hopes that the basic principles described above are accurate even though the exact or specific details may not be totally agreed upon by all of his professional colleagues, present and past.

Durrant, J. D., & Lovrinic, J. H. (1984). *Bases of hearing science* (2nd ed.). Baltimore: Williams & Wilkins.

Gelfand, S. A. (1997). *Hearing: An introduction to psychological and physiological acoustics* (3rd ed.). New York: Marcel Dekker.

Harris, J. D. (1986). *Anatomy and physiology of the peripheral auditory mechanism.* Austin, TX: Pro-Ed.

Kemp, D. T. (1978). Stimulated acoustic emissions from within the human auditory system. *Journal of the Acoustical Society of America, 64,* 1386–1391.

Moore, B. C. J. (1997). *An introduction to the psychology of hearing.* London: Academic Press.

Pickles, J. O. (1988). *An introduction to the physiology of hearing.* London: Academic Press.

Shaw, E. A. G. (1974). The external ear. In W. D. Keidel & W. D. Neff (Eds.), *Handbook of sensory physiology* (Vol. 5/1, pp. 455–490). Berlin: Springer.

Watson, J. D. (1968). *The double helix: A personal account of the discovery of the structure of DNA.* New York: Atheneum.

Yost, W. A. (1994). *Fundamentals of hearing: An introduction* (4th ed.). New York: Academic Press.

Zemlin, W. R. (1998). *Speech and hearing science: Anatomy and physiology* (4th ed.). Englewood Cliffs, NJ: Prentice-Hall.

CHAPTER

3

Contributions from the Psychoacoustics Research Laboratory

The author will not spend a great deal of time discussing this formal scientific background for clinical audiology. Thus, the student can relax and take a deep breath, because psychoacoustics is an extremely complex and extensive field of study that has resulted in a virtual mountain of very excellent beginning and advanced level textbooks that students can go read if they get bitten by the bug to do so. The behavioral test tools that audiologists have developed to test various aspects of human hearing have, of course, been borrowed from the field of psychoacoustics. The biggest difference between clinical audiology and psychoacoustics has to do with the amount of time that professionals in the two areas have at their disposal for getting the test results or information they need. The audiologist must operate under the gun of a very strict time limit and does not have the luxury of doing extensive and complex testing, lest he lose clinic revenues and his job. The audiologist must assess his patient's hearing status very quickly because his profession typically requires him to see many patients each day. The psychoacoustician, on the other hand, has the luxury of taking his time to do more extensive testing and collect more detailed information on the hearing status of only small numbers of experimental subjects or participants (scientists' term for the people they test, as contrasted to the audiologist's patient or client). Whereas the patient/client may need to be completely tested in a time frame of 30 minutes or less, the research subject may be tested for as much as an hour at a time, for several hours each day (with rest breaks between sessions to avoid fatigue or boredom), with perhaps the tests being repeated over a period involving several days. Thus, while the audiologist is forced to gather quick, cursory data that may not be as complete as he might like, the psychoacoustician can gather much more data and much more complex data, which allows a higher degree of scientific rigor. In the earlier part of his career, the author performed psychoacoustics tests with animals and humans. When he switched to being a clinical audiologist, it was very difficult to adjust to the need to work faster and settle for gathering less data in his new role as a clinician.

The author needs to implore the reader not to take his statements in the last paragraph too literally as meaning that audiologists, in doing quicker testing, are forced to perform less accurate testing. Fortunately, audiologists and hearing scientists (psychoacousticians) ask totally different questions. The kinds of questions (clinical) that the audiologist needs to answer require far less time and effort to answer. The hearing scientist typically asks extremely complex, basic science types of questions that require large amounts of data (information), which require more tedious testing procedures. It is, however, the obligation of the audiologist to keep eyes and ears open with respect to what the hearing scientist is doing, because the research findings of these people may provide critical information for development of different and more sensitive clinical test procedures.

Historically, the psychoacoustics laboratory has provided a significant amount of very important information about both the normal functions of the human auditory system as well as the procedures and techniques that must be utilized in the laboratory and the clinic to make test results accurate and reliable. The author strongly recommends that the reader find a good, introductory level textbook in psychoacoustics and read it very thoroughly to further enhance her understanding of this important scientific field.

Before leaving the present discussion of the scientific bases for clinical audiology, the author will briefly summarize the basic information that has emerged from the psychoacoustics laboratory related to how sensitive the human auditory system is to various types of sounds. This summary will only be a brief highlight of the more critical (from the standpoint of clinical audiology) aspects of normal human hearing.

Human Sensitivity to the
Basic Physical Parameters of Sound

The three physical properties or parameters of all air-conducted sounds are frequency, intensity, and the various temporal aspects of sounds. The human auditory system is most sensitive to frequency changes and least sensitive to the temporal aspects of sounds. With respect to frequency, the normal human ear can detect changes as small as 1 or 2 parts in 1000. This high level of sensitivity to frequency extends over a wide frequency range and a wide physical intensity range. It is only at frequencies close to the low (below about 125 Hz) and upper ends (at or above 8000 Hz) that this degree of sensitivity begins to decrease. This level of frequency sensitivity also tends to hold steady for most of the intensity range and only drops off for the very soft and very intense intensity levels. Thus, if presented with a 1000 Hz pure tone, most healthy young persons would be able to distinguish this tone from a tone of 1001 or 1002 (or 998 or 999) Hz. For many years, this degree of sensitivity came as a surprise to the hearing scientists. Most scientists believed the tonotopic organization of the BM was the source of the ear's sensitivity to frequency (see the author's earlier discussion of how the basilar membrane varies in stiffness from base to apex, which allows inner hair cells at different levels to fire in response to tones of different frequency). Several researchers, beginning with Georg von Bekesy in the 1950s (who was awarded a Nobel Prize for this work), drilled holes in the walls of the cochleas of animals and human cadavers and placed a camera inside to record the movement of the BM in response to sounds of different frequency. While these researchers saw evidence that the pattern of BM vibration does indeed reflect a tonotopic organization based on its inherent resonant frequency properties, the smoothness of this activity was far too gross to explain the exquisite sensitivity reported by behavioral testing. For many years, researchers searched without success for a "second filter" located somewhere in the brainstem or higher up in the nervous system where nerve cells acted to further refine the frequency information that was sent up from the cochlea. We now know that it is the outer hair cells that, in addition to extending the normal sensitivity range for intensity, somehow also "sharpen" the pattern of vibration of the BM to allow this increased sensitivity to frequency. Exactly how this is done is a very hot topic of investigation by many hearing scientists scattered across the globe.

To continue our discussion of the normal ear's capacities, the psychoacoustics laboratory folks also report that the ear is not quite as sensitive to changes in physical intensity as it is to frequency. The normal ear can detect only 1 or 2 parts per 100 (as contrasted to 1000 for frequency). For example, for a sound measured to be 50 dB SPL, most young adults would be able to detect a 0.5 or 1.0 dB change, e.g., from 50 to 50.5 or 51 (or 49 or 49.5) dB. As with frequency, this sensitivity holds over much of the normal hearing range and only begins to worsen at very soft and loud intensity levels and very low and high frequencies.

In contrast to intensity, the normal ear is 10 times less sensitive to changes in the temporal aspects of sounds. The human ear can detect changes only as small as 1 or 2 parts per 10. This is somewhat complicated by the fact that, in contrast to intensity and frequency, the temporal aspects of sounds come in a variety of different forms, including the rate of presentation of sounds, the length or duration of sound pulses, the physical location of sounds, and so on. Finally, related to the duration or length of sounds, it is also known that the normal auditory system takes a small but finite amount of time to process any incoming sounds. This process is not unlike the fixed amount of time that a camera lens needs to be opened to ensure optimal exposure of the film. This required processing time amounts to approximately 200 milliseconds (a millisecond is one one-millionth of a second). Thus, any sounds (regardless of frequency, complexity, or to some degree, intensity) that are shorter than 200 milliseconds in duration will not be perceived as accurately as longer sounds. Sounds, for example, that are 100 milliseconds in duration will not be perceived as intense (loud) as they would if longer. Also, tone pulses shorter than 200 milliseconds in duration would require a greater change in frequency before the normal listener could perceive the change. As is the case for both frequency and intensity, the sensitivity levels for the temporal aspects of sounds hold steady over a very wide range of the human audiogram.

Suggestions for Further Reading

Gelfand, S. A. (1997). *Hearing: An introduction to psychological and physiological acoustics* (3rd ed.). New York: Marcel Dekker.

Moore, B. C. J. (1997). *An introduction to the psychology of hearing*. London: Academic Press.

PART

II

What Audiologists Do and What You Need to Know

In this section of the text, the author will describe, again using as little technical jargon and as much layman's terminology as possible, what specific kinds of behavioral, electrophysiological, and physiological test procedures the audiologist uses to assess the nature of the patient's hearing problems, and determine where in the system (peripheral or central) the source of the problem is located. As stated earlier, the student who is preparing to become a practicing speech-language pathologist will not need to learn the specific procedures for each of the tests. However, some knowledge of how the tests are performed is needed to allow a fuller understanding of both the purpose and the results found with different tests. Since many of the patients that come to the SLP clinic may have hearing aids or other forms of assistive listening devices, the SLP will also need to know how to perform cursory checks or examinations of these devices to determine whether they appear to be in good working order or whether the patient needs to take them to the audiologist for detailed examination and possible repair or replacement.

4

Intake History and Otoscopic Examination of the Patient's Ear Canal and Eardrum

Both audiologists and speech-language pathologists are thoroughly trained and indoctrinated on the value of the intake history examination for providing insights into what the patient's problems may be and guiding the selection of specific test procedures. Most formal clinical evaluation reports prepared by audiologists contain a section related to the patient's recent medical history, possible family history (clues to genetic problems), recent episodes of hearing or dizziness problems, and current complaints or problems. The SLP must carefully read this section as it likely will provide information as to why the audiologist proceeded with the particular test protocol she chose. The SLP may choose to ask new questions to obtain additional information from the patient as it relates to specific problems with communication. In the written clinic report, the audiologist may report what she, or the referring otolaryngologist (ear, nose, and throat doctor), observed when examining the patient's ear canals with an otoscope. The otoscope is a small handheld device that has a small magnifying lens and a light that, when inserted into the patient's ear canal, allows the physician to view the ear canal and TM and see evidence of injury or disease (Figure 4–1). In today's

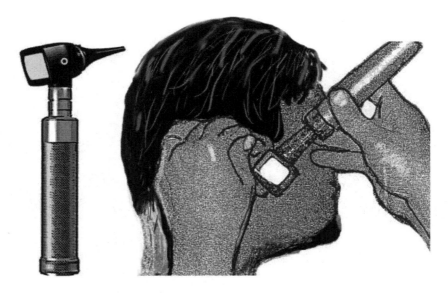

Figure 4–1. The otoscope is a small handheld device with a magnifying lens and light source that allows the physician or audiologist to view the ear canal and lateral aspects of the eardrum.

computerized medical world, many clinicians are beginning to take digital photos of the ear canal and eardrum. Patients may bring such photographs with them to the SLP clinic. Hopefully, however, the audiologist's report will have a written summary of what the photos show, because the typical SLP will not be expected to be able to interpret such photos by herself. Practicing SLPs will not be expected to perform otoscopic examinations, but they should be able to make sense of what is described in the audiologist's report.

In performing the otoscopic examination the audiologist or otolaryngologist will be looking for evidence of disease or injury. In the normal ear, the TM will appear somewhat blue or gray in color. In some patients, depending on the thickness of the TM (the thickness varies from patient to patient), the umbo of the malleus (the umbo is the point at which the malleus attaches to the TM) may be faintly visible behind the TM (Figure 4–2). The ear canal should be relatively clear of cerumen (earwax) or at least clear enough that the TM can be seen. If the canal is impacted with earwax, some small degree of conductive hearing loss may occur.

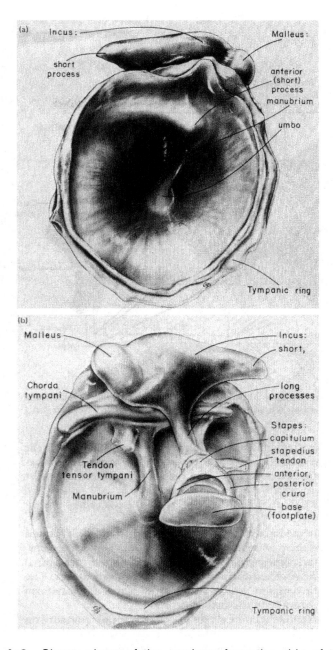

Figure 4–2. Shows views of the eardrum from the side of the ear canal (**A**) and from the inside of the middle ear space (**B**). Reproduced from *The Surgical Anatomy of the Temporal Bone and Ear* (p. 194), by B. J. Anson and J. A. Donaldson, Philadelphia: W. B. Saunders. Copyright 1967.

The audiologist or the otolaryngologist, but not the SLP, is author-ized (by scope of practice) to remove the cerumen, if needed.

The most common types of pathology that the audiologist may report in her report include the following.

Evidence of Tearing or Rupture of the TM

This type of injury could result from external sources (e.g., foreign objects being shoved into the canal) or from excessive positive (middle ear filled with fluid because of middle ear disease) or neg-ative (closing of eustachian tube resulting in absorption of air in middle ear space) air pressure. Depending on the location of the tear, some impairment of TM vibration may result. If the tear is located in a region that is normally tightly attached to the umbo of the malleus, some conductive hearing loss may result. If the tear is located in a region that is not tightly attached to the malleus, little hearing loss will result.

Evidence of Excessive Scar Tissue on the TM

If the TM has been repeatedly torn and healed in the past (perhaps due to repeated episodes of middle ear infections and repeated spontaneous ruptures), excessive amounts of scar tissue may be present. This changes the acoustical vibratory characteristics of the TM (makes it thicker and stiffer), which can result in some small degree of low frequency conductive hearing loss.

Evidence of Outward Bulging or Inward Retraction of TM

Outward bulging indicates the middle ear space is partially or completely filled with fluid as a result of middle ear pathology. A retracted eardrum indicates the middle ear space has been closed off (closure of eustachian tube) and the air in the middle ear space has been partially absorbed by the mucous membrane lining to cre-ate a partial vacuum. In the normal course of middle ear infections, the retraction symptoms typically precede those of the TM bulging.

Both bulging and retraction of the TM will alter the vibratory characteristics of the TM, making it stiffer, which tends to partially block transmission of lower frequency sounds.

Evidence of Blood behind the TM

This finding usually indicates some kind of traumatic injury (e.g., head blow) that has caused a rupturing of some blood vessels located in the middle ear space.

Evidence of Injury or Pathology of the Ear Canal

The audiologist may see evidence that the ear canal may have been torn or injured by foreign objects, or she may see evidence of other pathologies such as neoplasms (abnormal growths of tissue, whether cancerous or benign) or skin lesions (e.g., swimmer's ear infections).

CHAPTER

5

Pure Tone Air and Bone Conduction Audiometry— How to Interpret the Patient's Audiogram

The auditory system of the average young adult is sensitive to sounds from approximately 10–15 Hz (at the lower frequencies, the patient may feel vibrations rather than hear sounds) at the low frequency end of the audiometric scale to close to 20,000 Hz at the high frequency end. However, since virtually all of the critical speech information (for the different consonants and vowels) occurs in the frequency range from close to 250 Hz to 4000 Hz (see Figure 2–4B), audiologists only test hearing sensitivity for the frequencies of 125, 250, 500, 1000, 2000, 4000, and 8000 Hz. To conserve time in the busy audiology clinic, the audiologist measures thresholds for only these seven frequencies because they encompass the critical frequency range for a human's most important hearing function, i.e., verbal speech communication. If time allows, the audiologist may also test at other in-between frequencies such as 750, 1500, or 3000 Hz to get a more complete picture of a particular patient's hearing loss. This additional information may assist the clinician in more accurately fitting the patient with hearing aids. It needs to be mentioned that, if the physician suspects that a patient (for example, a cancer patient) may be in danger of having ototoxic reactions to certain drug treatments, he may ask the audiologist to test at frequencies above 8000 Hz. Hearing loss due to ototoxicity tends to occur first at the higher frequencies (between 8000 and 20,000 Hz). If the audiologist sees evidence for the beginnings of a hearing loss at the higher frequencies, he may alert the physician who may, in turn, alter the treatment regimen for the patient.

The patient's hearing sensitivity at each of the seven basic audiometric frequencies is reported in the form of a special chart known as the audiogram. Each of the seven different frequencies is plotted along the horizontal axis of this chart, while the patient's threshold levels are plotted along the vertical axis. Hearing threshold levels at each frequency are measured using the earlier mentioned (see discussion of decibel) hearing level or HL scale. In reporting the results of their clinical testing of patients, audiologists utilize a formal written audiogram format which allows the collection of data not only of pure-tone thresholds, but also middle ear function (tympanograms, to be discussed later), acoustic reflexes, and speech discrimination/detection. Figure 5–1 shows the format of the audiogram sheet used in the author's speech and hearing clinic at the LSU Health Sciences Center. As indicated earlier, the human ear is not equally sensitive to all frequencies. Of the audiometric range of test frequencies, the ear is least sensitive to 125 Hz and 8000 Hz and most sensitive to the mid-frequencies of 1000 and 2000 Hz. If you measured the average young adult's threshold using the dB SPL scale, you would get the results shown in Table 5–1.

As mentioned earlier, the HL scale was developed by audiologists to simplify the task of reporting the threshold levels exhibited by patients at different audiometric frequencies. This was accomplished by adjusting the internal circuits of the audiometer to compensate for the inherent normal differences in sensitivity. In order for the 0 dB HL level on the dial of the audiometer to reflect the same average human detection threshold for each frequency, the base amplitude (i.e., the lowest intensity that average young humans can detect) of different frequencies had to be set at different levels. Since the average ear is most sensitive to 1000 Hz (which, at threshold, is measured to be 7.5 dB SPL), this frequency was made the base level or standard around which the intensity levels of the other lower and higher frequencies were set.

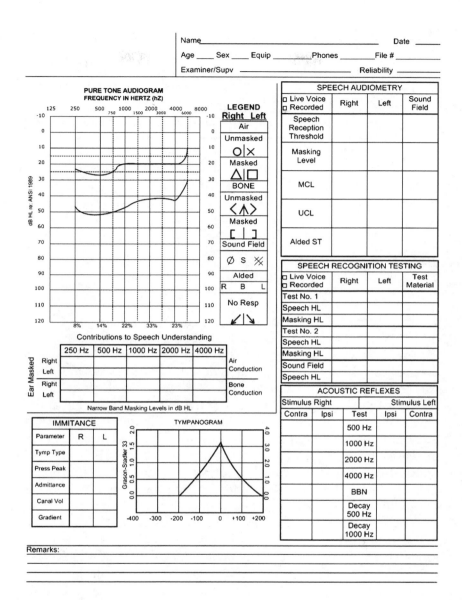

Figure 5–1. Shows the format of the basic clinical audiogram along with the symbols used to depict various aspects of the testing, such as air versus bone conduction testing, use of masking, and position of the earphone or bone vibrator. Most audiogram report forms depict test results for not only air and bone threshold testing, but all the other test procedures (acoustic reflex tests, speech discrimination tests, and tympanometry). The form shown is the one used in the author's audiology clinic at LSU Health Sciences Center.

Table 5–1. Comparison of average hearing thresholds for healthy young adults as measured with the sound pressure level (SPL) versus the modified hearing level (HL) method used by audiologists

TEST FREQUENCY	SPL THRESHOLD	HL THRESHOLD
125 Hz	45 dB	0 dB
250 Hz	27 dB	0 dB
500 Hz	13.5 dB	0 dB
1000 Hz	7.5 dB	0 dB
2000 Hz	9 dB	0 dB
4000 Hz	12 dB	0 dB
8000 Hz	15.5 dB	0 dB

Thus, the intensity level of the 125 Hz circuit was set to be 37.5 dB more intense, 250 Hz was set to 17.5 dB more intense, 500 Hz was 6 dB more intense, 2000 Hz was 1.5 dB more intense, 4000 Hz was boosted by 4.5 dB, and 8000 Hz was raised 8 dB higher. As indicated earlier, the different HL threshold levels are plotted along the vertical axis of the audiogram. The least intense levels are plotted at the top of the axis and the most intense at the bottom. The typical audiogram starts with the lowest intensity level of −10 dB HL, then increases in 5 dB steps (−5, 0, 5, 10, etc.) to the most intense level (loudest or most intense sounds) of 100 or sometimes 110 dB HL. The greater an individual patient's hearing loss, the lower on the scale will the threshold level be plotted. It is important to note that, although 0 dB HL is considered to be the threshold of the average young adult, some people (and especially children) may be more sensitive and, thus, the need to include levels of −5 or −10 dB HL. For clinical purposes, healthy adults (persons in their late teens or greater) are considered to have *clinically normal* hearing if their thresholds fall at or below 25 dB HL. With children, some audiologists will want to see levels of 20 dB HL or lower before concluding that the child has normal sensitivity. In terms of their ability to communicate, the audiologist considers a pure tone average threshold (PTA at frequencies of 500, 1000, and 2000 Hz, which are in the middle of the speech spectrum) of 26 to 40 dB HL to be a *mild* loss, 41 to 55 dB HL to be *moderate,* 56 to 70 dB HL to be *moderately severe,* whereas 71 to 90 dB is a *severe* loss. Anything greater than 91 is considered *profound* (Martin & Clark, 2000).

The audiologist performs two forms of pure-tone threshold tests. The first are air-conducted threshold tests. These tests examine the integrity of the entire system from the ear canal, through the middle ear space, to the point at which nerve impulses begin to travel out of the cochlea into the brainstem. Sounds are presented directly using specially calibrated headphones that fit over the pinna, or more frequently in recent years, using specially calibrated insert earphones or transducers that are inserted into the ear canal, not unlike ear plugs. Problems at any point in the peripheral system that impede the transmission of vibratory energy will result in an apparent loss of hearing sensitivity: excessive cerumen in the ear canal, absent or collapsed ear canals, ruptured, scarred, or stiffened TMs (due to negative middle ear pressure or presence of middle ear fluids), disruption of the ossicular chain, fixation of the stapes in the oval window (due to otosclerosis), or even stiffness due to excessive inner ear fluid (caused by Ménière's disease). The air-conducted test will also show evidence of hearing loss if the inner or outer hair cells are damaged or missing or malfunctioning in any way.

If the audiologist suspects that the cause of the patient's apparent hearing loss is due to disruption of one or more of the conductive portions of the peripheral system, but does not involve the inner hair cells, he may perform the second special form of threshold test, known as a bone-conducted threshold test. Figure 5–2 depicts the difference between air- and bone-conducted testing. With this test, the audiologist places a small calibrated mechanical vibrator snugly on the patient's head (with a small amount of calibrated pressure against the skin produced by a metal headband), usually behind the ear over the mastoid part of the skull, or sometimes in the middle of the forehead. The vibration from this bone vibrator is then transmitted to the bone of the patient's skull. The skull tends to vibrate as a unit, which includes vibration of the mastoid bone region that directly surrounds the cochlea. This vibratory disturbance in the mastoid bone is then transmitted to the perilymph of the cochlea, where it proceeds to produce the subsequent events (upward and downward movement of the basilar membrane, shearing of the stereocilia of the inner hair cells) that lead to the generation of nerve impulses. It is important to note that the pattern of vibration of the perilymph is essentially the same whether it results from the inward and outward shoving of the stapes at the oval window or to the vibration of the surrounding mastoid bone. If the bone-conducted thresholds are found to be normal, but the air-conducted thresholds

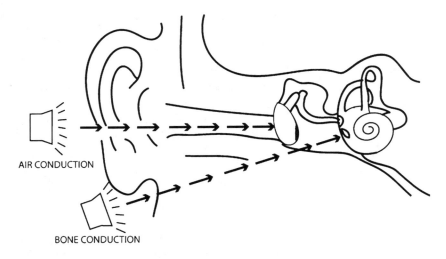

AIR CONDUCTION

BONE CONDUCTION

Figure 5–2. Depicts the pathways by which air and bone vibrations reach the inner ear. Whereas the air conduction route involves transferring vibrations from the eardrum through the ossicles to the stapes and oval window, the bone conduction route bypasses these structures and directly elicits vibrations of the entire skull, which are then transferred to the fluid contents (perilymph) of the cochlea.

indicate the presence of a hearing loss, this indicates the patient has a conductive hearing loss and not a sensory hearing loss. With the conductive form of hearing loss, the patient probably has a problem with one or more of the peripheral stages involving transmission of vibratory energy. The presence of normal bone conduction thresholds suggests that the sensory portion of the system involving the hair cells is working properly. Normal air-conducted thresholds in conjunction with lowered bone conduction thresholds should not be present if the audiometer is working properly. However, it is possible for patients to have mixed hearing losses in which parts of the conductive system as well as the hair cells are both malfunctioning.

The author will now summarize the basic kinds of audiometric findings that will most likely appear in typical audiograms.

Normal Hearing Sensitivity

Most audiologists consider the adult patient's hearing to be clinically within normal limits when the pure tone thresholds are 25 dB HL or better at both ears for all frequencies from 125 Hz to 8000 Hz. The same patient's bone conduction thresholds at frequencies from 250 to 4000 Hz should be close (within ± 5 dB of the air conduction scores, 5 dB being considered the maximum chance deviation that typically occurs in audiometric testing) to the air conduction scores. Of course, as indicated earlier, some young children and young adults may exhibit scores better than 20 dB HL (e.g., at 10, 5, 0, or even below 0 at –5 or –10). It is important to note that, because of physical limitations related to the nature of bone conduction testing, the audiologist never tests bone thresholds at 125 or 8000 Hz, since these scores would probably not be accurate. Figure 5–3 shows a normal audiogram obtained from a patient.

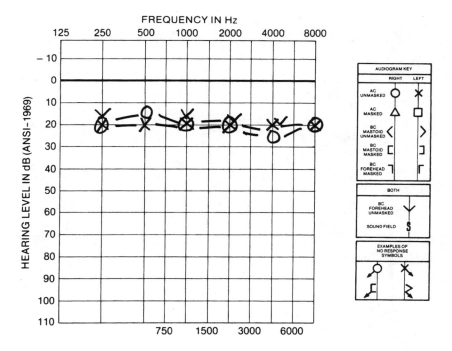

Figure 5–3. Audiogram showing normal hearing sensitivity in both ears. The air and unmasked bone conduction thresholds are in good agreement at about 20 dB HL. Thresholds of 25 dB HL or lower are considered normal for adults, but many audiologists will want to see lower thresholds (10 dB HL or better) for young children, whose sensitivity is frequently better than that of adults.

Sensory Hearing Loss

This is a hearing loss involving some kind of problem related to the elicitation of normal neural impulses by the inner hair cells. The most common variety of sensorineural hearing losses involves loss of outer hair cells due to noise exposure, aging, or intake of some form of ototoxic chemical (e.g., antibiotics). Since this type of loss involves pathology of the hair cells, the patient's bone conduction thresholds will also exhibit evidence of a hearing loss and should agree closely (± 5 dB) in threshold level with those obtained with air conduction testing. Figure 5–4, Figure 5–5, Figure 5–6, and Figure 5–7 show a series of audiograms from patients with sensory hearing losses in one or both ears.

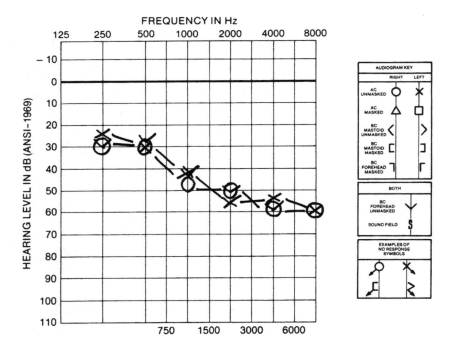

Figure 5–4. Audiogram showing sensorineural hearing loss in both ears. The unmasked bone conduction thresholds are in close agreement with the air-conducted thresholds. This patient exhibited mild difficulty at both ears in hearing the high frequency consonant sounds with the word discrimination test.

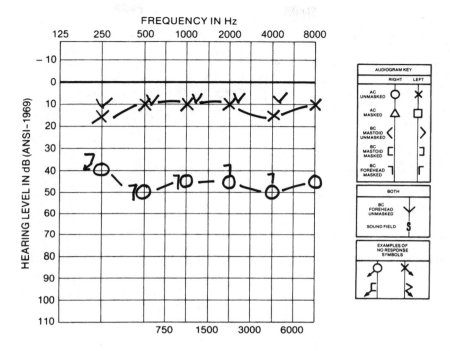

Figure 5–5. Audiogram showing normal air and bone thresholds in the left ear. The unmasked bone conduction thresholds obtained with a forehead placement were in close agreement with the left ear air conduction thresholds. In contrast, air conduction testing in the right ear shows the presence of a hearing loss at all frequencies. Air conduction testing of the right ear was performed with masking noise presented through a bone vibrator placed on the forehead. This masked test procedure indicated the hearing loss in the right ear is sensorineural in nature.

Conductive Hearing Loss

With this type of hearing loss, the inner hair cells (and outer hair cells) are functioning appropriately, but there exists a problem at some lower level that is impeding the normal vibratory transmission of sound energies to the cochlea. Air-conducted testing will show hearing losses at some or all frequencies, depending on the location of the problem and what specific changes in the natural resonant frequency characteristics of the peripheral system have

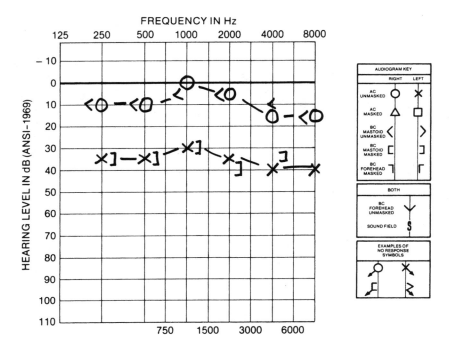

Figure 5–6. Air-conducted testing suggested the presence of normal sensory function in the right ear combined with a hearing loss in the left ear. Unmasked bone conduction tests were in good agreement with the right ear threshold tests. Since unmasked bone conduction tests always agree with the better or more sensitive ear results (in this case, the right ear), the audiologist measured masked bone conduction thresholds. These masked bone conduction results were close to that of the left ear air conduction results, indicating the loss in the left ear was sensorineural in nature.

occurred. The most common variety of conductive hearing loss involves the lower frequencies of 500 Hz and below. This is due to the fact that the most common varieties of conduction problems involve an overall stiffening of the system, which impedes the transmission of low frequency sounds more than high frequency sounds. With pure conductive hearing losses, the bone conduction thresholds will be in the normal range or at least better than the air conduction thresholds, at the different affected frequencies (lower

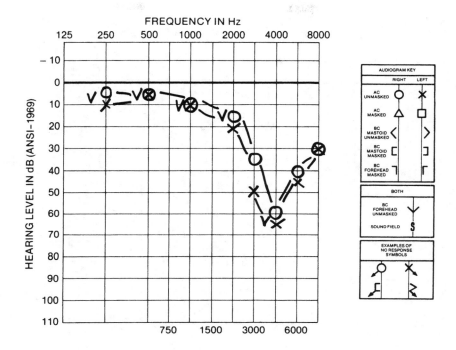

Figure 5–7. Audiogram showing typical results from a patient who has a long history of noise exposure. Air conduction and unmasked bone conduction results are in close agreement at all test frequencies, confirming the loss to be sensory in nature. This patient exhibited moderate levels of difficulty at both ears hearing the high frequency components of the word discrimination test.

frequencies, most typically). Figure 5–8, Figure 5–9, and Figure 5–10 show test results from different patients with conductive hearing losses in one or both ears.

Mixed Sensorineural and Conductive Hearing Loss

Many older patients, as well as younger people who have lived especially active lifestyles (attended lots of loud rock concerts, consumed taboo recreational chemicals that poisoned their outer hair cells) or have an inherited or genetic form of hearing loss, may exhibit a combination of both air conduction and bone conduction

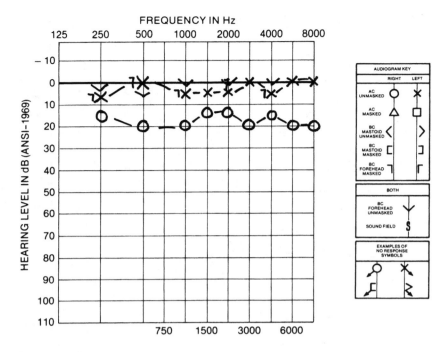

Figure 5–8. Audiogram showing a mild conductive loss in the right ear with normal thresholds in the left ear. Although unmasked bone tests agree with the better (left) ear air conduction test results, with the left ear masked, the bone conduction thresholds stay in agreement with unmasked results, indicating the loss in the right ear is conductive. It is important to note that, in this patient, air conduction thresholds are clinically normal (20 dB HL or better) at both ears, even though there is an interaural asymmetry. This interaural asymmetry is a cause of concern for the audiologist because it may signal the development of a hearing problem, and the patient will need to be monitored.

hearing loss. These mixed losses are frequently more difficult for the audiologist to evaluate behaviorally and report, which as a consequence also makes them more difficult for the SLP practitioner to understand and interpret. In the next paragraph, your author will describe, as painlessly as possible, how the audiologist tackles the difficult task of discerning which ear may be suffering more from a hearing loss, and also whether it involves a simple sensory or con-

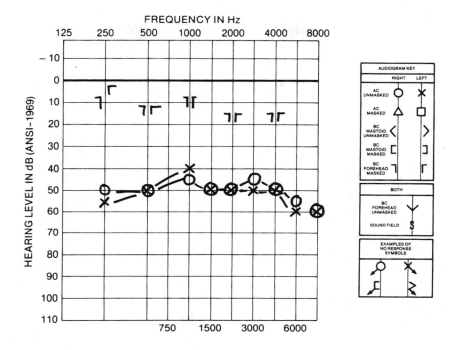

Figure 5–9. Audiogram showing a moderate conductive hearing loss in both ears. Whereas air conduction thresholds are 55 dB HL or worse at all frequencies in both ears, masked bone conduction at both ears is well in the normal range from 5 to 15 dB HL, confirming the loss to be conductive in nature. This patient had severe otitis media affecting both middle ear systems.

ductive loss or a more complicated mixed hearing loss. Figure 5–11 and Figure 5–12 show test results from two patients who have mixed sensory and conductive hearing losses.

The "Agony" of the Audiological Evaluation of Mixed Hearing Losses

As the reader by now has begun to realize, the auditory system of humans is not a simple entity but is a very complex association of many different subsystems (peripheral vs. central, sensory vs.

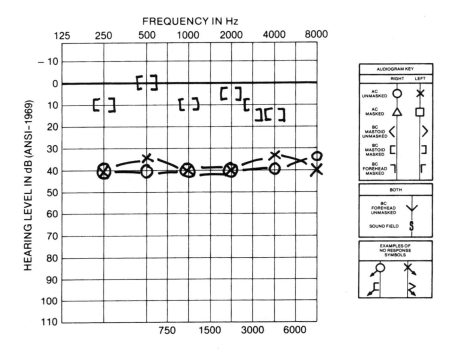

Figure 5–10. A second example of an audiogram illustrating bilateral conductive hearing loss. Unlike the example shown in Figure 5–9, this test was performed with the bone oscillator placed on the mastoid rather than the forehead. With bone conduction testing, it makes little difference whether the bone vibrator is placed on the forehead or on the mastoid, as the entire skull vibrates equally well with both placements. With unmasked bone testing, the amount of vibration that arrives at one cochlea is virtually identical whether the bone vibrator is placed on the ipsilateral or contralateral mastoid site.

conductive, etc.) that all must work together in order for its owner to hear appropriately. Because a person has two ears, the audiologist must test each ear separately. If the patient has any kind of hearing loss, it will be necessary for the audiologist to amplify the sounds to more intense levels in order to identify the patient's threshold levels. The existence of the phenomenon of bone conduction (the fact that intense sounds delivered via vibrating air molecules will cause not only the TM and middle ear components to vibrate, but will also

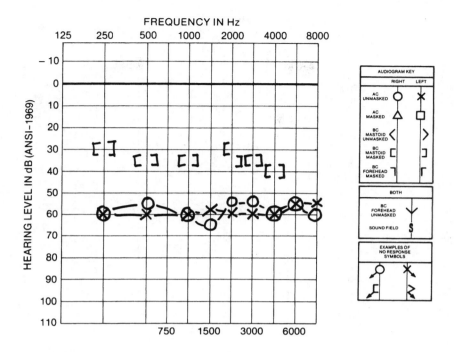

Figure 5–11. Audiogram showing a mixed sensory and conductive hearing loss in both ears. The air conduction thresholds range between 55 and 65 dB HL, but the masked bone conduction thresholds range from 20 to 40 dB HL. Thus, part of the total hearing loss of approximately 60 dB HL is due to an inner ear sensory problem, but the rest is the result of a problem somewhere in the conductive portion of the system.

cause the whole skull and temporal bone to vibrate) creates a real problem for the audiologist. At intensity levels above about 40 or 50 dB HL, when stimuli are presented by circumaural headphones, the entire skull will begin vibrating and the amount of the vibration may be sufficient for the cochlea on the other side of the head (non-test ear) to be stimulated. The opposite ear may, therefore, be able to eavesdrop or listen in on the sounds being presented to the test ear. If the patient responds to this bone-conducted sound, it may completely invalidate the audiologist's test findings. The recent switch by the profession to using insert earphones has decreased

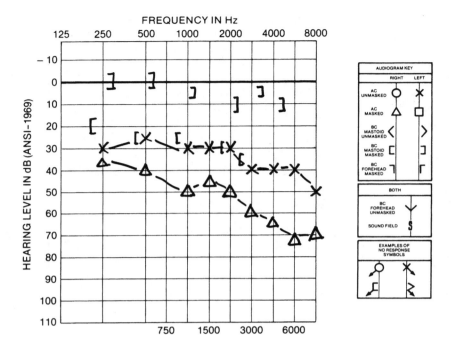

Figure 5–12. Audiogram showing a mixed sensory and conductive hearing loss in the right ear and a purely conductive loss in the left ear. Masking was required for both air and bone conduction tests to resolve the nature of the loss in the right ear.

this problem, because these phones can actually increase the interaural attenuation of this unwanted bone conducted "leakage" to levels of 60 or 70 dB HL. The use of insert phones also eliminates the problem of the circumaural phones causing a collapsing of the pinna/ear canal, which results in a conductive hearing loss. This latter problem occurs most often in elderly patients and some younger children. However, as many older individuals, or patients with severe noise or ototoxic exposure, may have threshold levels higher than 60 or 70 dB HL, it is necessary for the audiologist to take steps to ensure that the non-test ear cannot listen in on what is being presented to the test ear. The non-test ear must be "kept busy" at all times while the other ear is being tested.

The way the audiologist does this is to present continuous masking noise to the opposite ear throughout the duration of the testing. Broadband masking noise (or "white" noise) is a complex mixture of all the different pure tone frequencies (or sine wave components) that covers the entire frequency range that the normal ear is sensitive to (not unlike white light, which is a mixture of all the colors of the rainbow that the eye is sensitive to). Since broadband noise is perceived as loud and annoying, as a result of containing all the different frequencies, what the audiologist actually uses is band-limited noise (sometimes referred to as narrowband noise or NBS) that contains fewer frequencies and is less annoying but just as effective at keeping the ear busy. When testing each tonal frequency, what the audiologist does is continuously present a signal that contains a limited range of frequencies centered around the test frequency (the noise is turned on all the time and is perceived as steady and unchanging). For example, if testing at 1000 Hz, the noise in the opposite ear would be the immediate adjacent frequencies above and below 1000 Hz (800 to 1200 Hz).

When the patient's detection thresholds appear to be in the "danger zone" where there is a risk that the loud tones might be able to be inadvertently perceived by the opposite non-test ear, the audiologist will switch to using masking noise and measure the patient's masked air and bone conduction thresholds. Audiology students, as a critical part of their training, receive extensive training and practice in using a number of clinically approved (approved for clinical use by the American Speech-Language-Hearing Association) masking protocols to allow them to accurately determine which ear has which form of hearing loss and at what severity levels. SLP students can relax at this point, knowing that they will not need to learn how to do this themselves, but they will need to know what masking is and what is used for and, most importantly, how to read and interpret the audiologist's complex audiometric test results. SLP students should not thumb their noses at their audiology student colleagues but instead send them flowers (or a case of beer) as a gesture of sympathy for their having to tackle this tough task of masking. Masking and the decibel are two of the biggest headaches that audiology students must encounter in the classroom and clinic. Figure 5–6, Figure 5–7, Figure 5–9, Figure 5–10, Figure 5–11, and Figure 5–12 depict different audiograms in which masking was used to identify the true nature of the patients' hearing loss.

References and Suggestions for Further Reading

Dirks, D. D. (1994). Bone-conduction threshold testing. In J. Katz (Ed.), *Handbook of clinical audiology* (4th ed., pp. 132–146). Baltimore: Williams & Wilkins.

Gelfand, S. A. (1997). *Essentials of audiology*. New York: Thieme.

Keith, R. W. (1996). The audiologic evaluation. In J. L. Northern (Ed.), *Hearing disorders* (3rd ed., pp. 45–56). Needham Heights, MA: Allyn and Bacon.

Martin, F. N., & Clark, J. G. (2000). *Introduction to audiology*. Boston: Allyn and Bacon.

Yantis, P. A. (1994). Puretone air-conduction threshold testing. In J. Katz (Ed.), *Handbook of clinical audiology* (4th ed., pp. 97–108), Baltimore: Williams & Wilkins.

CHAPTER

6

Speech Audiometry: What It Can and Cannot Reveal about Peripheral versus Central Auditory Function

In addition to air- and bone-conducted pure tone threshold tests, the basic audiometric evaluation also includes assessing the patient's ability to detect and understand speech sounds. Two forms of tests are used. One test, known as the speech reception threshold (SRT), measures how loud speech sounds have to be in order for the patient to be able to understand them (verbally recite them back to the examiner). Special lists of spondee words have been developed for this purpose. These consist of two-syllable words such as *baseball*, *cowboy*, and *hotdog* that are either spoken by the examiner (using a sound level meter to monitor and control her own voice level) or from a commercially available recorded list (for example, Auditec). The words are presented first at levels below threshold and are then increased in intensity level (5 dB steps) until the patient begins to correctly repeat them back. The intensity level at which the patient first begins accurately repeating the words is taken as the SRT. In normal patients, the SRT level should lie relatively close to the pure tone thresholds in the mid-frequency range (e.g., 1000 and 2000 Hz).

The second form of speech test is known as the word discrimination test (or WDS for short). For this purpose, special lists of 25 or 50 phonetically balanced (PB) (monosyllabic or single syllable) words have been developed. PB word lists contain all of the different phonemes (basic speech sounds) of the language and in the same relative proportions that occur in normal, everyday speech. The word lists are presented either orally by the audiologist or in a tape-recorded or CD format. Since this test is designed to assess the ability of the patient to understand normal conversational speech, the lists are presented at levels 30 to 40 dB above the patient's SRT threshold level.

Patients with relatively normal pure tone air-conducted thresholds from 500 to 4000 Hz should have no difficulty performing the two speech tests. Persons who have severe high frequency sensory hearing loss may not perform as well on the SRT and WDS tests because of the inability to distinguish certain consonant sounds. Also, persons with conductive hearing losses may have difficulty with these tests if the stimuli are delivered by air conduction but probably not if delivered by bone conduction. However, any patient whose SRTs or WDS results are poorer than would be expected based on the pure tone thresholds may have a central auditory processing problem, which suggests some form of pathology at higher levels of the auditory nervous system. Figures 5–4 and 5–7 show two examples of audiograms in which the patients exhibited problems with the word discrimination test.

References and Suggestions for Further Reading

Jerger, J., & Hayes, D. (1977). Diagnostic speech audiometry. *Archives of Otolaryngology*, *103*, 216–222.
Martin, M. (Ed.). (1997). *Speech audiometry* (2nd ed.). San Diego, CA: Singular.

CHAPTER

7

What Are Acoustic Reflexes and What Do They Reveal about the Patient's Auditory Function

The stapes is the smallest of the three middle ear ossicles. As indicated earlier, it is shaped like the stirrup of a saddle. The footplate of the stapes sits directly on top of the small oval window membrane. When the stapes moves in and out, it transmits vibratory energy that causes pressure changes in the perilymph of the inner ear. Attached to the side of the stapes is a small striated muscle, the other end of which is attached to the wall of the middle ear space. This stapedius muscle is the smallest striated muscle in the human body (Figure 7–1). When it contracts, the muscle pulls the stapes laterally, which acts to slightly reduce the amount of the shoving action of the stapes footplate against the oval window. This allows a small amount of protection against loud, steady background noise but provides no protection against sudden loud sounds such as gunshots. This is because the reflex action of the stapedius muscle to sudden loud sounds is too slow to allow it to contract in time to offer protection. Thus, while factory workers may gain some benefit from this tiny muscle, hunters do not. However, similar to the piston action of the outer hair cells, the contraction of the stapedius

AUDITORY OSSICLES – Ligaments and Muscles

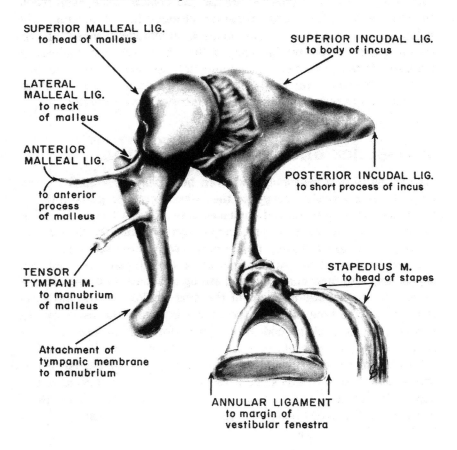

Figure 7–1. Depicts the normal ossicular chain of the middle ear along with the attached ligaments and muscles. See text for functional details. *Reproduced from Surgical Anatomy of the Temporal Bone and Ear* (p. 245), by B. J. Anson and J. A. Donaldson, Philadelphia: W. B. Saunders. Copyright 1967.

muscle produces vibratory energy that can travel back out through the ossicles and TM and be detected as small pressure changes in the air-filled ear canal. The acoustic reflex is an automatic neural reflex to sudden sounds and has nothing to do with any higher perceptual processes in the brain. Audiologists can measure the acoustic reflex and measure its properties as another tool for determining whether the peripheral parts of the auditory system are healthy.

When loud sounds are presented to just one ear, the stapedial muscles in both ears will elicit a contraction. Thus, the audiologist can measure the integrity of the patient's uncrossed and crossed stapedial reflexes, by inserting measuring devices (sensitive microphones) in either the ear receiving the sounds or in the opposite ear. Figure 7–2 depicts the equipment used to test crossed and uncrossed acoustic reflexes. The acoustic reflex usually does not occur unless the sound is relatively loud, at least 85 dB or more above the patient's threshold. Thus, the absence of acoustic reflexes may confirm the existence of a number of different forms of hearing loss (severe sensory and conductive as well as mixed losses). The absence of ipsilateral reflexes even at the limits (intensity) of the equipment may indicate either a severe cochlear (sensory) hearing loss or some form of pathology involving the 8th cranial nerve (such as acoustic neuroma). The absence of crossed reflexes in the presence of uncrossed or ipsilateral reflexes suggests some form of pathology in the lower brainstem where the nerve fibers for the crossed reflex arc are located. Figure 7–3, Figure 7–4, Figure 7–5, and Figure 7–6 show examples of reflex testing where patients exhibit normal (in the range of 85 dB HL) or abnormal (elevated or absent) crossed and uncrossed acoustic reflexes. Also shown in these figures are the tympanogram results, which will be discussed in the next section.

If the audiologist suspects pathology at the level of the 8th cranial nerve or at the level of the lower brainstem, he may administer a special acoustic reflex decay test. A lower frequency tone (either 500 or 1000 Hz) is presented continuously for a period of 10 seconds at a level that is 10 dB greater than the patient's acoustic reflex threshold. In normal individuals, the onset of this tone will elicit the acoustic reflex and the reflex contraction will be maintained during the whole 10 second time period. If it is elicited but is not maintained (it *decays*), this suggests an 8th nerve or brainstem problem.

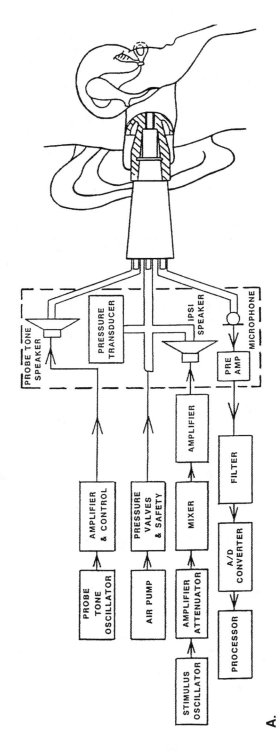

Figure 7–2. (A) Shows a schematic drawing of the electroacoustic immittance meter used in tympanometry testing as well as acoustic reflex tests (Courtesy of Grason-Stadler, Inc.). *continues*

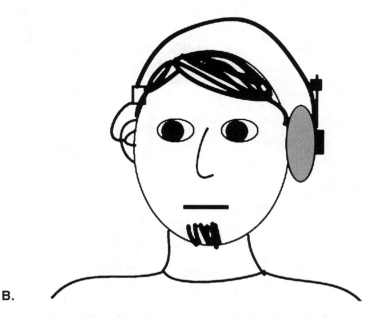

B.

Figure 7–2. *continued* **(B)** With contralateral (crossed) acoustic reflexes, the sound source (tones) are presented by an earphone (or insert phone) placed on the opposite ear, whereas with ipsilateral acoustic reflex testing as well as tympanometry, everything is done through the immittance meter (changing air pressure for tympanometry testing, or presenting tones for acoustic reflex tests).

ACOUSTIC REFLEXES

Frequency (Hz)	RIGHT				LEFT			
	500	1000	2000	4000	500	1000	2000	4000
Ipsilateral (Probe same)		90	90			95	100	
Contralateral (Probe opposite)	95	90	95	100	85	85	90	90
Audiometric Threshold	50	45	50	55	5	5	0	10
Reflex SL	45	45	40	40	80	85	90	85
Decay Time (Seconds)	10+	10+			10+	10+		

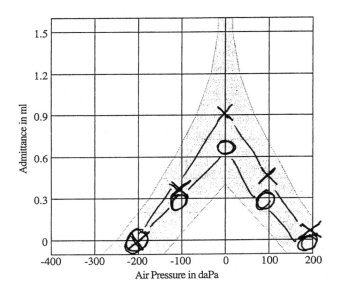

Figure 7–3. Acoustic reflexes (top of figure) and tympanograms (bottom graph) recorded from patient with Ménière's disease in the right ear. This problem results from the presence of excess amounts of endolymph in the scala media of the cochlea, which causes a stiffening of the inner ear function. This is evidenced by the lower point of compliance of the right ear relative to the left ear in the tympanogram and slightly increased reflex thresholds in the right ear.

ACOUSTIC REFLEXES

Frequency (Hz)	RIGHT				LEFT			
	500	1000	2000	4000	500	1000	2000	4000
Ipsilateral (Probe same)		*NR*	*NR*			95	90	
Contralateral (Probe opposite)	*NR*	*NR*	*NR*	*NR*	*NR*	*NR*	*NR*	*NR*
Audiometric Threshold								
Reflex SL								
Decay Time (Seconds)								

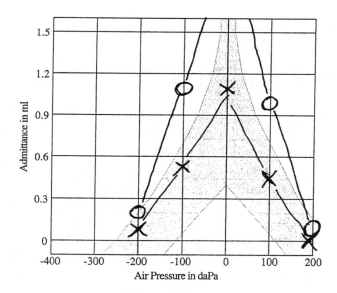

Figure 7–4. Acoustic reflexes and tympanograms recorded from a patient exhibiting abnormally decreased stiffness of the right middle ear system. The compliance of the left ear is within normal limits. This patient's problem is due to a discontinuity of the ossicular chain in the left ear that resulted from a traumatic blow to the right side of the head in a motorcycle accident.

ACOUSTIC REFLEXES

Frequency (Hz)	RIGHT				LEFT			
	500	1000	2000	4000	500	1000	2000	4000
Ipsilateral (Probe same)		90	85			NR	NR	
Contralateral (Probe opposite)	80	80	80	85	NR	NR	NR	NR
Audiometric Threshold	5	0	0	5				
Reflex SL	75	80	85	75				
Decay Time (Seconds)	10+	10+						

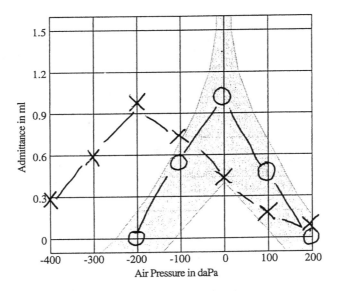

Figure 7–5. Acoustic reflexes and tympanograms showing abnormal negative pressure in the left ear combined with normal middle ear pressure in the right ear. This problem is frequently associated with transient middle ear disease related to allergy problems or otitis media.

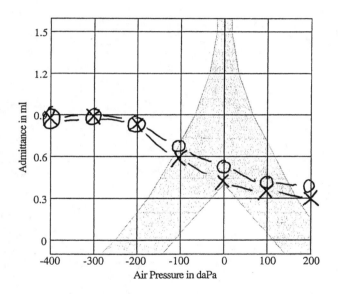

ACOUSTIC REFLEXES

Frequency (Hz)	RIGHT				LEFT			
	500	1000	2000	4000	500	1000	2000	4000
Ipsilateral (Probe same)		NR	NR			NR	NR	
Contralateral (Probe opposite)	NR	NR	NR	NR	NR	NR	NR	NR
Audiometric Threshold								
Reflex SL								
Decay Time (Seconds)								

Figure 7–6. This "flat" (absence of a discernible peak in either ear) tympanogram indicates the presence of more severe otitis media involving either negative pressure or the accumulation of middle ear fluid in both ears. Acoustic reflexes were absent in both ears.

Suggestions for Further Reading

Fowler, C. G., & Wiley, T. L. (1997). *Acoustic immittance measures in clinical audiology.* San Diego, CA: Singular.

Northern, J. L. (1996). Acoustic immittance measurements. In J. L. Northern (Ed.), *Hearing disorders* (3rd ed., pp. 57–72). Boston: Allyn and Bacon.

CHAPTER

8

Tympanometry and Tympanograms: What They Reveal about the Patient's Middle Ear Function and Hearing Status

As discussed earlier, the major function of the middle ear system is to overcome the normal hearing loss that would occur if sound, which starts as vibrating air molecules, had to directly produce vibrations in the inner ear fluid-filled space. Fluid is denser and stiffer than air, and this *impedance mismatch* would result in only about 1% of the energy from the air being transmitted into the fluid medium with 99% being reflected away and lost. In order for the middle ear to do its job and overcome this impedance mismatch, all of the structures of the middle ear (the TM, the ossicular chain, and also the ambient air pressure of the middle ear chamber) must maintain normal density and stiffness characteristics. If this changes for any of the structures (e.g., eardrum becomes stiffer due to scarring, negative middle ear air pressure, or fluid behind the TM; the ossicular chain becomes discontinuous due to trauma), the entire system will take on a different natural resonant frequency property that will alter the normal transmission of sounds into the inner ear space. Depending on the nature of the changes and which structures are involved, mild, moderate, or severe conductive hearing losses for different frequencies will result.

Tympanometry is a tool used by the audiologist to measure changes in the normal compliance of the middle ear system. *Compliance* is a term borrowed from the science of physics, which indicates how stiff a system is and how easily it can be bent or have its shape altered by external forces. During tympanometric testing, a special probe is placed in the external ear canal (see Figure 7–2A). The fit of the probe has to be tight enough to completely seal the air-filled space between the tip of the probe and the TM from the outside world. The probe is designed to do two things. First, air is pumped into the sealed-off space to increase the ambient air pressure to a high level. Next, the air pressure is gradually decreased until it reaches the same level as the outside world, and then more air is pumped out to gradually produce a partial vacuum. As the air pressure in the sealed-off space is gradually changed from higher to lower levels, a continuous low frequency probe tone (either 220 or 226 Hz) is elicited from the probe tip in the direction of the TM. The probe contains a small microphone that continually measures the amount of the probe tone that is reflected back from the TM. Per our earlier discussion of the relationship between natural resonant frequency and the transmission of sound from one medium to another, it is expected that the least amount of sound will be bounced back (the TM will vibrate most easily) when the air pressure below the probe and that on the other side of the TM are equal. As the pressure on the probe side becomes either greater or less than the pressure in the middle ear space, more and more of the tonal energy will be bounced back and recorded by the probe microphone.

Today's tympanometric equipment generates and prints out a special chart, known as the tympanogram. Figure 8–1 shows the five most common types of normal and abnormal tympanograms that are typically found with various forms of middle ear dysfunction. The air pressure changes are plotted on the horizontal axis of this chart, ranging from negative pressure (partial vacuum) on the left, through ambient pressure (normal sea level pressure) in the middle, to positive increased pressure on the right. Depicted on the vertical axis are the changing compliance or stiffness levels of the TM, as measured by how easily the TM vibrates (transmits the energy of the probe tone to the middle ear) as the air pressure on

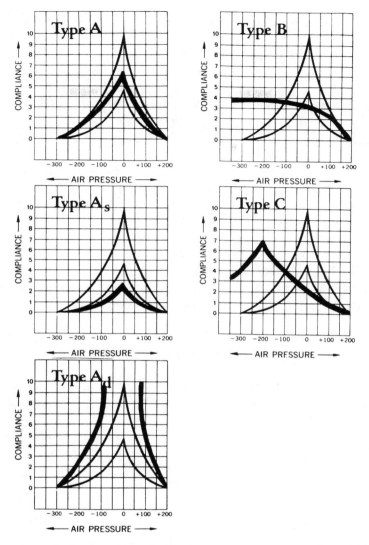

Figure 8–1. Summary of the five most common varieties of normal and abnormal tympanograms typically found in patients. Definition of pathology types: *Type A* – Normal middle ear (ME) stiffness; *Type B* – Severe increased ME stiffness, due to negative air pressure and/or fluid behind eardrum; *Type C* – Increased ME stiffness, similar to Type B but less severe; *As* – Increased ME stiffness, possibly due to scarring of eardrum or fixation of ossicular chain; *Ad* – Decreased ME stiffness due to torn or ruptured eardrum which prevents obtaining any evidence of a pressure peak with the test equipment. Reproduced with permission from *Hearing in Children* (3rd ed., p. 184), by J. L. Northern and M. P. Downs, Baltimore: Williams & Wilkins. Copyright 1984.

95

the probe side changes. The combined position (on the horizontal axis) and the height (on the vertical axis) of the resulting peak of the tympanogram tracing indicate how stiff or noncompliant the middle ear system has become. For example, if the patient has a middle ear infection and has negative air pressure in the middle ear space, the peak of the tympanogram will be located to the left side of the chart directly above the negative air pressure portion of the horizontal axis. If the eardrum is very stiff (perhaps due to severe TM scarring, fixation and nonmovement of the ossicular chain, or thick mucus filling the middle ear space), the tympanogram will be flat with no discernible peak. If, on the other hand, the TM is badly torn and moves more easily than usual, the peak will be in the middle of the horizontal axis (indicating normal sea level pressure on both sides of the TM) but very high or off the chart. If the peak of the tympanogram falls close to 0 air pressure and entirely within the shaded area, the result is considered normal (Type A).

Suggestions for Further Reading

Stach, B. A., & Jerger, J. F. (1991). Immittance measures in auditory disorders. In J. T. Jacobson & J. L. Northern (Eds.), *Diagnostic audiology* (pp. 113–140). Austin, TX: Pro-Ed.

Electrocochleography and Brainstem Auditory Evoked Potential Tests and What They Reveal about Auditory Functions

In the late 1970s, with the advent of inexpensive digital computers, audiologists were able to develop the first of what has become a series of extremely valuable nonbehavioral tools for evaluating the physiological integrity of the peripheral and brainstem components of the auditory nervous system. The first procedure, which was discovered in the early 1970s, involves measuring the electrical activity of the cochlea and lower brainstem portions of the system when sounds are presented to the ears. These tests involved placing recording electrodes (not unlike those used to record EKG or EEG activity) behind the ear on the mastoid area and on the scalp, typically at the vertex or top of the head. Sounds, typically continuous trains of repeating clicks or brief duration tone pulses, are presented to the ear with circumaural or insert phones and the resulting electrical activity of the brain is recorded. With the electrocochleography (or ECOG test), the recording electrode is placed deep in the ear canal in close proximity to the tympanic membrane. The closeness of this electrode to the inner ear and 8th cranial nerve allows it to record the electrical activity in the cochlea that immediately precedes (i.e., the cochlear microphonic and summating potentials) the elicitation of action potentials by the inner hair cells. The ECOG test can, therefore, be used by the audiologist to evaluate the functional status of the cochlea and 8th cranial nerve. Abnormalities in the ECOG recordings can be used to identify cochlear disease processes such as Ménière's disease (a disease that involves the presence of excessive amounts of endolymph in the scala media).

With the more widely used auditory brainstem response (or ABR test), the placement of the recording electrode on the vertex of the scalp (or sometimes high forehead) allows the recording of activity that occurs in the lower (where the 8th nerve inserts) and upper parts of the auditory brainstem pathways and neural centers (Figure 9–1). It is important to note that neither of these tests reveals anything about the patient's ability to consciously hear or perceive sounds, which is the job of the higher portions of the auditory nervous system (midbrain and cortex). The recordings are unaffected by the patient's level of consciousness. Sleeping or fully awake patients show the same responses. Even patients with severe cortical damage (due to strokes or head injuries) who are in a coma state exhibit normal ECOGs and ABRs. The audiologist uses these tests to evaluate the neurological integrity of these lower parts of the system. Abnormal or absent ECOGs or ABRs can occur as a result of a number of pathological conditions in the cochlea (such as Ménière's disease, or loss of inner hair cells) and brainstem (strokes, traumatic injury, or acoustic neuromas, sometimes referred to as acoustic or 8th cranial nerve tumors or acoustic schwannomas). In recent years, the ABR test has become a very important tool for evaluating hearing sensitivity in newborn infants. Growing numbers of medical centers have instituted programs to screen all newborns who are determined to be at high risk for hearing loss due to prematurity, family history, or other medical problems. The ABR, while not a direct test of hearing, can assess the neural integrity of the critical neural structures (cochlea and brainstem) that are a prerequisite for normal hearing. Any infant who fails the newborn ABR screen is not assumed to have a hearing problem but is brought back for further testing to rule it out.

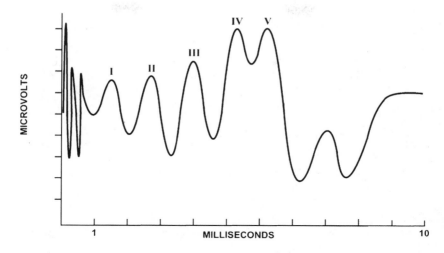

Figure 9–1. Shows an example of a typical auditory brainstem response (ABR) recorded from a normal young adult. Because the ABR is a subcortical response, it exhibits very reliable and repeatable latencies and amplitudes of its positive and negative waveforms. This makes it a very useful clinical tool for evaluating the physiological status of the lower portions of the auditory nervous system.

Suggestions for Further Reading

Glattke, T. J. (1983). *Short-latency auditory evoked potentials: Fundamental bases and clinical applications.* Baltimore: University Park Press.

Hall, J. W., III. (1992). *Handbook of auditory evoked responses.* Boston: Allyn and Bacon.

Hood, L. J. (1998). *Clinical applications of the auditory brainstem response.* San Diego, CA: Singular.

10

Otoacoustic Emissions: The Latest Computerized Tool for Assessing Peripheral Hearing and Neural Function

As indicated earlier, the outer hair cells in the cochlea have a unique motor function that acts to increase the magnitude of the basilar membrane vibration (and resulting shearing of the stereocilia of the sensory inner hair cells) when less intense sounds are being presented to the ear. The outer hair cells, which are ironically shaped like pistons, begin to elongate and shorten and increase the magnitude of the vibration of the overhanging tectorial membrane. In essence, the outer hair cells begin to vibrate. The vibratory energy of the outer hair cells travels out through the structures of the cochlea, through the oval window, and cause the TM to vibrate. If a special probe that contains a sensitive microphone is inserted into the ear canal, it will be able to pick up the vibrations coming from the outer hair cells. These vibrations can then be analyzed by the audiologist to determine if they are "normal" and indicate the outer hair cells, and presumably the other structures of the cochlea, are functioning appropriately. These so-called *otoacoustic emissions* (OAEs), depicted in Figure 10–1, can be recorded in normal infants

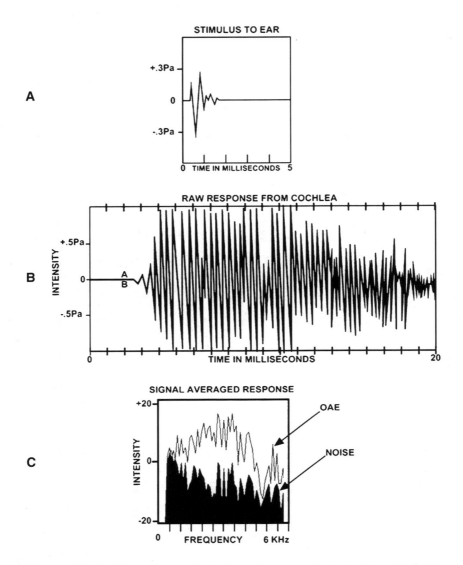

Figure 10–1. When the outer hair cells are activated, they begin to alternately elongate and shorten and push on the tectorial membrane. These vibrations of the outer hair cells can be picked up and recorded by small recording devices placed in the canal close to the eardrum. The characteristics of these vibrations, or otoacoustic emissions (OAEs), can be examined to determine whether the outer hair cells are functioning appropriately or not. (**A**) Shows the waveform of the click stimulus that is presented to the ear. (**B**) Depicts the response coming back from the cochlea. (**C**) After computerized signal averaging, the OAE response can be seen above the noise background.

and adults as long as they have relatively normal hearing sensitivity (threshold levels at or below 30 dB HL). A growing number of audiologists are beginning to use the recordings of OAEs as another tool (in addition to the auditory brainstem response) for screening newborn hearing status. One form of otoacousitc emissions, known as the distortion product OAE (DPOAE), can even detect the normal distortion that occurs when the healthy cochlea is "overdriven" by louder sounds.

Suggestions for Further Reading

Robinetdte, M. S., & Glattke, T. J. (1997). *Otoacoustic emissions: Clinical applications.* New York: Thieme.

CHAPTER

11

Common Forms of Behavioral Assessments Used by Audiologists to Assess Central Auditory Function

As indicated earlier in the present text, while we know a great deal about the anatomy, physiology, and functions of the peripheral auditory nervous system (outer, middle, and inner ear), we know far less about the higher (brainstem, midbrain, and cortical levels) centers of the system. However, thanks to the efforts of large and divergent groups of neuroscientists, neurologists, and experimental psychologists over the past 100 or more years, a lot of new information has been gathered, some of which has led to the development of behavioral tools that can distinguish between pathologies at the peripheral versus central levels of the system. Some of these tests have also been found to provide information about the spatial location of the problems in the system (whether brainstem or higher cortical centers). In this chapter, the author will summarize some of the more reliable and clinically useful tests that have been developed that the SLP may encounter in some of the audiologists' clinical reports. These test procedures are frequently referred to as central auditory processing (CAP) or central auditory nervous system

(CANS) tests. In the earlier part of his career, the author performed and published animal model studies and research with patients with CANS lesions and made a significant contribution to this field of study.

During the early part of the 20th century a number of audiologists in this country (Jerger & Jerger, 1975) and in Italy (Bocca, Calearo, & Cassinari, 1954; Bocca, Calearo, Cassinari, & Migliavacca, 1955) and Russia (Karaseva, 1972) made the important discovery that patients with lesions of the higher cortical centers (like the temporal lobe) of the auditory system had much more difficulty than persons without lesions in discriminating various kinds of sounds that had been physically altered in some manner to make them harder to understand. If sounds are presented in a difficult listening situation, such as a noisy room, everyone has more difficulty perceiving them. However, patients who have temporal lobe pathology were found to perform much more poorly than normal individuals. A number of formal central test procedures have been developed that can be utilized in the clinic to identify persons who have difficulty understanding speech in the presence of competing noise. A widely used example of this type of speech-in-noise test is the speech-perception-in-noise or SPIN test developed by Kalikow, Stevens, and Elliott (1977). Other researchers (see Musiek & Baran, 1987, for a good review of this literature) found that, if the physical or acoustical parameters of normal sounds (such as taped recordings of spoken words) were altered, while normal persons had perceptual difficulties, the difficulty levels of temporal lobe patients was markedly exaggerated. Some of the common acoustical alterations that were investigated included filtering out some of the frequency information contained in normal spoken words (frequently referred to as the filtered speech test). This was accomplished by passing the words through special electronic filters so that only some of the normal frequency content was retained in the recording. A second commonly used test (known as the altered speech rate test) presented the spoken words (or sentences) at faster or even slower rates than normal to the two ears. Another test involved presenting part of the spoken word to one ear and the second part to the other ear (for example, using two-syllable words like *cowboy* or *hotdog* and presenting *cow* or *hot* to the left ear followed by *boy* or *dog* to the right ear). This test was known as the alternating or swinging speech test. In the real world, both syllables would normally be presented to both ears. In essence, all of these tests were designed to reduce the normal redundancy that occurs with normal spoken speech. It appears that, when the higher cortical centers of the auditory system are damaged, the lack of redundancy in normally spoken words becomes a major handicap for the patient.

Perhaps the most frequently used version of the alternating or swinging speech test is the Staggered Spondaic Word (SSW) test developed by audiologist and hearing scientist, Dr. Richard Katz (1962). This test is used and reported often enough that the practicing SLP may see it described in some audiological evaluation reports. As indicated above, the spondaic word is a special type of two-syllable word (*cowboy*, *hotdog*, *baseball*) that is used when performing speech reception threshold (SRT) testing. Katz developed an ingenious test that presents two different spondaic words to the patient's two ears in a partially overlapping (or temporally "staggered") manner. For example, if one spondaic word is *racehorse* and the other word is *streetcar*, they would be presented to the two ears in the following manner:

Ear 1   race   horse

Ear 2   street   car

Thus, ear 1 would receive the two consecutive *race* and *horse* syllables, while ear 2 would receive *street* followed by *car*. The two spondaic words would be presented in a temporally staggered manner so that *horse* and *street* would be presented at the same time. The SSW test has been shown to be sensitive to the presence of a variety of different pathologies involving the central auditory neural pathways. Whereas many normal adults (and children) will be able to accurately report both spondaic words, some may suppress and fail to report different parts of the complex stimulus. For example, because of CANS pathology, the patient may fail to hear the two competing components (*horse* and *street*) and only report back the word *racecar*. Others may completely suppress the stimuli at one ear and only report back what they heard at the other ear (such as only reporting back *racehorse* or *streetcar*, but not both). Over the years, Dr. Katz and his students and colleagues have obtained research evidence that suggests that particular types of error patterns on the SSW test may be associated with different forms or location of neural pathology. The referring audiologist should in his report elaborate not only on the nature of the abnormal findings obtained with the SSW test, but also summarize what the findings indicate related to the specific nature of the patient's problems.

The author has also developed a CANS test procedure that reveals the sensitivity of the impaired central auditory system to sounds that are reduced in their normal stimulus redundancy. In the earlier psychoacoustics section of the text, the author indicated that the normal auditory system requires a minimum of approximately 200 milliseconds (0.2 seconds) to complete the normal analysis or processing of incoming sounds. Tone pulses that are shorter than approximately 0.2 seconds in duration are not perceived to be as loud as longer sounds. Also, the smallest frequency change that can be detected (the frequency difference limen or threshold) is also elevated. Thus, sounds shorter than approximately 0.2 seconds are not long enough to allow the normal auditory nervous system to completely process them before they are turned off. The author (Cranford, 1984) has found that many elderly listeners and patients with various forms of central auditory system pathology (such as temporal lobe lesions, multiple sclerosis) break down much more on this brief tone discrimination test than do normal persons. The effect seems to be more severe for the frequency difference limen portion of the test than it is for the loudness portion. For 1000 Hz tones with durations of 20 milliseconds (0.02 seconds), although normal individuals show frequency difference thresholds of 15 to 30 Hz, some elderly and patients with impaired temporal lobes may exhibit thresholds as high as 150 Hz or more (remember, for longer tones, the normal threshold may be as small as 1 or 2 Hz). It is interesting that, whereas elderly listeners show this effect in both ears, patients with damaged temporal lobes show it only for the ears located contralateral to the side of the cortical lesion.

A recent study by the author (Allen, Cranford, & Pay, 1996) found evidence that whether or not patients with temporal lobe lesions exhibit problems discriminating brief tones, may be dependent on the age at which the lesion occurred. Figure 11–1 shows test results with a patient (left graph) who was born with an absent left temporal lobe and a patient (right graph) that suffered the lesion as an adult. This finding suggests that, because of neural plasticity, the brain can compensate for injuries sustained early in life (before puberty).

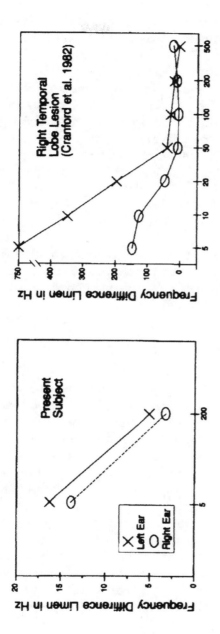

DURATION IN MSEC

Figure 11–1. When tone pulses are shorter than approximately 200 milliseconds (0.2 of a second) in length, normal persons require larger differences in frequency in order to tell them apart than when they are 200 ms or longer. The normal auditory nervous system apparently requires at least 200 ms of stimulation in order to have time to completely analyze the sound. Some patients with temporal lobe lesions (and some elderly persons) require even greater frequency differences in order to detect the change. Reproduced with permission from "Central auditory processing in an adult with congenital absence of left temporal lobe," by R. L. Allen et al., 1996, *Journal of American Academy of Audiology, 7,* pp. 282–288.

Thus, it appears that the higher centers of the auditory system are unusually sensitive to both reduced redundancy in the normal stimulus content of sounds as well the presence of stimulus competition at the two ears. One additional test, developed by Dr. Frank Musiek (Baran & Musiek, 1991), shows this competition effect. This dichotic digits test is very similar to the SSW, but rather than using spondaic words, it uses digits (numbers) from 1 to 9 (excluding the two-syllable number seven). Two digits are presented to each ear in a partially overlapping fashion, which, like the SSW, involves the second digit of one ear overlapping in time with the first digit of the other ear. Normal listeners can usually report back all four digits. However, patients with auditory cortical lesions exhibit problems perceiving the two digits that are presented in a competing manner to the two ears.

Before leaving the topic of tests of central auditory pathology, the author will describe two more test procedures that have been found to be valuable in identifying CANS dysfunction. In addition to having difficulty understanding competing sounds or sounds that have been distorted in some manner (such as filtered or placed in noise), many patients with CANS lesions also exhibit difficulties perceiving many of the normal temporal aspects of normal sounds. The ability to locate where sounds are coming from requires the nervous system to analyze small differences in the time of arrival or loudness of sounds at the two ears. We now know, from both animal studies and studies with neurological patients, that pathology located at the cortical level can disturb the patient's ability to accurately locate the source of sounds. The author's earlier research with animals (Cranford & Oberholtzer, 1978) and patients with temporal lobe damage (Moore, Cranford, & Rahn, 1990) found that complex forms of sound localization tests are even more sensitive than simple localization tests for identifying central pathology. In this test of stereophonic listening (also known as the *precedence effect* phenomenon in sound localization), instead of locating the source of unitary sounds, patients are required to identify (or in one test version, track with a laser light pointer) the location of a fused auditory image (FAI) which is produced when the same sounds are presented from two spatially separated loudspeakers, but with one source leading the other by a very small amount of time (less than 1 millisecond). Figure 11–2 shows results found in the author's laboratory from a normal young listener and a patient with a right-

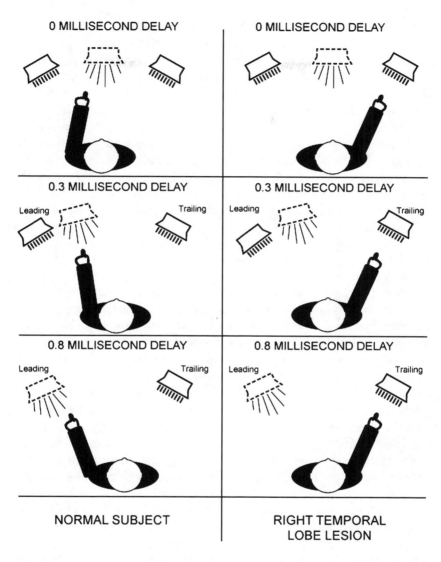

Figure 11–2. This illustrates the effects of unilateral auditory cortex lesions on a complex form of sound localization involving the precedence effect phenomenon. See text for details

sided temporal lobe lesion. Normal individuals can readily locate the source of the FAI (the "phantom" sound) resulting from presenting sound from two physically separated sound sources at the same time or with one speaker leading the other by a few thousandths of a second. When the leading speaker is located contralateral to the intact or undamaged hemisphere, normal listeners respond appropriately. However, when the leading speaker is located contralateral to the damaged hemisphere, patients with unilateral auditory cortex lesions respond as though the fused auditory image was originating from the speaker located opposite the intact hemisphere (they point to this side). This test, while a test of sound localization, is similar to the SSW and dichotic digits tests, since it too involves the presentation of competing sounds at the two ears. It is interesting to note that the patient described earlier (Allen et al., 1996) who was born with a missing left temporal hemisphere did not exhibit any problems with the precedence effect test.

The pathological effect observed with the author's stereophonic listening test (and perhaps also with the SSW and dichotic digits tests) reflects a more generalized neurological phenomenon sometimes referred to as sensory extinction or sensory inattention. This phenomenon was first reported by Dr. Hughlings Jackson, an eminent neurologist who practiced in Boston during the late 1800s. Jackson reported the same extinction effects with lesions located in the auditory cortical regions as well as other sensory systems such as somatosensory cortex and the visual cortical areas. Patients with unilateral somatosensory cortex lesions were not able to perceive a stimulus (such as a touch, rubbing of a feather, etc.) to the arm located contralateral to the cortical lesion when the other arm was also being stimulated at the same time in a similar fashion. In some cases involving more extensive unilateral cortical damage, the patients dressed only one side of their bodies in the morning (put a shoe on only one foot, placed only one leg into their trousers).

A second commonly used form of temporal processing test was developed by Dr. Frank Musiek and his students/colleagues in the mid-1980s (Baran & Musiek, 1991). Two versions of this test are available. Both involve testing the ability of patients to perceive the temporal order or temporal pattern of a series of three consecutive tonal stimuli. In the frequency pattern test, the patient is presented with three consecutive tones in which the frequency pattern varies. High and low frequency tones are presented in various combinations, for example, with patterns such as high-low-high (HLH), low-high-low (LHL), low-low-high (LLH), high-high-low (HHL), and the patient is required to verbally report back the specific sequence he hears (HLH, LHL). With the frequency pattern test, all of the tone pulses are equal in length. In a second duration pattern test, while the frequency of all tones is the same, the temporal duration (length) of the tones is varied, with some being short and some long, for example long-long-short (LLS), long-short-long (LSL), short-long-long (SLL). Children and adults with lesions or pathology involving the auditory cortex exhibit problems perceiving both kinds of pattern changes.

References and Suggestions for Further Reading

Allen, R. L., Cranford, J. L., & Pay, N. (1996). Central auditory processing in an adult with congenital absence of left temporal lobe. *Journal of the American Academy of Audiology, 7,* 282–288.

Baran, J. A., & Musiek, F. E. (1991). Behavioral assessment of the central auditory nervous system. In W. F. Rintelmann (Ed.), *Hearing assessment* (pp. 549–602). Austin, TX: Pro-Ed.

Bocca, E., Calearo, C., & Cassinari, V. (1954). A new method for testing hearing in temporal lobe tumors. *Acta Otolaryngologica, 44,* 210–221.

Bocca, E., Calearo, C., Cassinari, V., & Migliavacca, F. (1955). Testing cortical hearing in temporal lobe tumors. *Acta Otolaryngologica, 42,* 280–304.

Cranford, J. L. (1984). Brief tone detection and discrimination tests in clinical audiology with emphasis on their use in central nervous system lesions. *Seminars in Hearing, 5,* 263–275.

Cranford, J. L., & Oberholtzer, M. (1978). Role of neocortex in binaural hearing in the cat. II. The "precedence effect" in sound localization. *Brain Research, 111,* 225–240.

Cranford, J. L., Stream, R. W., Rye, C. V., & Slade, T. L. (1982). Detection versus discrimination of brief durations: Findings in patients with temporal lobe damage. *Archives of Otolaryngology, 108,* 1616–1619.

Jerger, J., & Jerger, S. (1975). Clinical validity of central auditory tests. *Scandinavian Audiology, 4,* 147–163.

Kalikow, D. N., Stevens, K. N., & Elliott, L. L. (1977). Development of a test of speech intelligibility in noise using sentence materials and controlled word predictability. *Journal of the Acoustical Society of America, 61,* 1337–1351.

Karaseva, T. A. (1972). The role of the temporal lobe in human auditory perception. *Neuropsychologia, 10,* 227–231.

Katz, R. E. (1962). The use of staggered spondaic words for assessing the integrity of the central auditory system. *Journal of Auditory Research, 2,* 327–337.

Moore, C. A., Cranford, J. L., & Rahn, A. (1990). Tracking of a "moving" fused auditory image under conditions that elicit the precedence effect. *Journal of Speech and Hearing Research, 33,* 141–148.

Musiek, F. E., & Baran, J. A. (1987). Central auditory assessment: Thirty years of change and challenge. *Ear and Hearing, 8*(Suppl.), 22–35.

Musiek, F. E., & Lamb, L. (1994). Central auditory assessment: An overview. In J. Katz (Ed.), *Handbook of clinical audiology* (pp. 197–211). Baltimore: Williams & Wilkins.

Recent Advances in Electrophysiology Measurement Tools for Assessing Central Auditory Nervous System Problems

Neurophysiologists are able to record electrical activity from all levels of the auditory nervous system and not just the cochlea (ECOG) and brainstem levels (ABR). In fact, electrical activity from higher levels of the brain is much larger in amplitude and easier to record than ABRs or ECOGs because the recording electrodes are located closer to the sources of the activity (that is, the cortex, which is located just below the skull, rather than deep subcortical centers such as the brainstem). However, this ease of testing of higher level activity is confounded by the fact that higher level activity (cortical) in the normal brain is much more variable and unpredictable than that from lower centers (brainstem). This is because the higher centers are involved in much more complex and constantly changing stimulus processing, including conscious perception, than are the lower centers. The ABR response is very stable. It is independent of the level of consciousness of the patient and looks the same regardless of whether the patient is awake or asleep or even in a coma. The latencies and amplitudes of the different peaks of the ABR recordings can be relied on to provide accurate indicators of changes in underlying neural functions. Small changes in the latencies of the ABR peaks can be used to identify the presence of severe pathology of the brainstem neural centers and pathways. Such is not the case with responses from the higher neural centers.

Figure 12–1 depicts the more commonly tested higher level responses that the SLP professional may encounter in the audiologist's reports. The middle latency response occurs immediately following the ABR and probably reflects neural activities at the level of the midbrain, thalamus, or auditory cortex. The next commonly recorded response is the late latency response (LLR), which is thought to reflect activity at the level of the auditory cortex. Finally, in recent years, a number of investigators have begun recording even later responses which are thought to reflect higher level cognitive processing at the level of the cortex and hippocampus (the memory centers of the brain). One of these responses, which is labeled the P300 response (named because it typically occurs about 300 milliseconds or 0.3 seconds after the sounds are presented), is thought to reflect the patient's active attention to and processing of the sounds. Another response, which occurs just before the P300, has attracted a lot of attention from neuropsychologists in recent years because it is believed to reflect the brain's unconscious monitoring of stimulus changes in the environment. This response is known as the mismatch negativity response.

Although not unexpected, it is clinically unfortunate that the amplitude or latencies of all of these later occurring responses vary greatly in normal individuals, and even in the same patients from one test session to another. These higher level responses are so "clinically flaky" that the presence or absence of the response may be the only useful indicator of normal or abnormal underlying neural function.

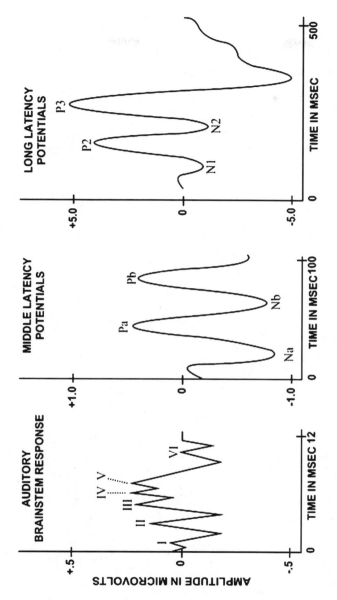

Figure 12–1. In recent years, clinical researchers have begun looking at evoked responses from the central parts of the auditory nervous system as a possible tool for diagnosing higher level auditory processing problems. While these responses are larger and easier to record than the lower level ABR response, the latencies and amplitudes of the different waves are typically quite variable, which makes them unreliable as indices of normal/abnormal function. Whether the waveform is present or absent is frequently the only valid clinical clue that can be used for diagnostic purposes.

Suggestions for Further Reading

Cranford, J. L., & Hymel, M. (1998). Pros and cons of brain mapping as a tool for investigating central auditory pathology. *Seminars in Hearing, 19,* 345–355.

Hall, J. W., III. (1992). *Handbook of auditory evoked responses.* Boston: Allyn and Bacon.

McPherson, D. L. (1996). *Late potentials of the auditory system.* San Diego, CA: Singular.

Naatanen, R. (1995). The mismatch negativity: A powerful tool for cognitive neuroscience. *Ear and Hearing, 16,* 6–18.

13

Use of Medical Neuroimaging Techniques to Assist in Evaluating CNS Problems in Patients

The emergence of inexpensive digital computer technology in the mid to late 1970s has launched a virtual (no pun intended) revolution in all of the medical diagnostics arenas. This technology is revolutionizing all areas of the biological and medical sciences, including audiology and speech-language pathology. Audiological measures of tympanometry, auditory brainstem response testing, and otoacoustic emissions are just the beginning of many new diagnostic tools that can be expected to emerge in the not too distant future. Unfortunately, the diagnosis of pathologies is far beyond our ability to come up with viable treatments or cures. We can now look inside the body (without disturbing the patient's tranquility) and can see what the problem is, but we may still not be able to do anything about it.

Since both audiology and speech-language pathology are brain sciences, the new neural imaging techniques are especially important for us. The marriage of computers and traditional x-ray technology occurred first during the late 1960s, to give us computerized tomography (CT scans), also known as computerized axial tomography (CAT scans). This technique allowed the radiologist, using the computer, to rapidly take a large number (series) of x-rays at multiple levels (hence the term *axial*) through the brain, and later to put them together as a three-dimensional composite. The CAT scan allowed the physician to better visualize the size and extent of any lesion (neoplasm, traumatic injury, stroke) that might be affecting the patient's brain.

By the beginning of the 1970s, a totally new neuroimaging technology emerged on the medical scene. Rather than x-rays, this new technique involved the realignment of hydrogen atoms using changing magnetic fields. The procedure, therefore, became known as magnetic resonance imaging (or MRI). With this technique, the patient's head (or whole body) is placed in a large, barrel-like structure, which contains a large magnet that completely surrounds the head. Hydrogen atoms are the predominant ingredient of the water molecule, H_2O, and water is the most common component of most tissues, including brain tissue. The water content of the different tissues in the brain (blood, myelin sheaths, fibers) varies and, thus, the amount of water content (and hydrogen) varies. The surrounding bone (skull) contains even less water. When the magnet is turned on it causes the normally random alignment pattern of the hydrogen atoms to suddenly realign together in the same direction. When the magnet is then turned off, each hydrogen atom "announces its presence" by emitting a signal (somewhat akin to gamma rays) that can be picked up and recorded by special instruments. During the test session, the magnet is continually turned on and off to allow the development of a "picture" that represents extremely small deviations in the hydrogen content in different regions of the brain and surrounding tissues. The turning on and off of the magnet is very noisy and many patients have to wear acoustic earplugs to reduce the annoyance. Some patients are also claustrophobic and do not like being stuck in a small enclosed space. In more recent years, the newer MRI systems have dumped the barrel concept and moved to "open space" systems that eliminate this problem. Figure 13–1 shows a MRI obtained from a very unusual patient tested in the author's laboratory who had a congenital absence of the left cortical hemisphere (Allen, Cranford, & Pay, 1996).

Today's MRI systems are becoming more and more sensitive, and the tests are becoming less expensive to administer. This tech-

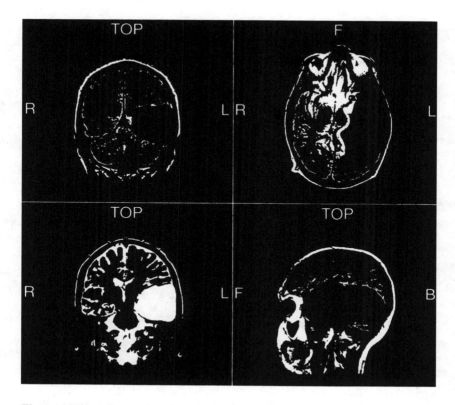

Figure 13–1. Example of magnetic resonance imaging (MRI) findings from a patient tested in the author's hearing research laboratory. This patient was born with an absent right cortical hemisphere. At 34 years of age, we presented this patient with a series of central auditory processing tests and discovered that the remaining left hemisphere had assumed all functions that normally would require both hemispheres working together to perform. This case is a remarkable example of the degree to which neural plasticity or compensation can occur when pathologies occur very early in life. See text for more details. Reproduced with permission from "Central auditory processing in an adult with congenital absence of left temporal lobe," by R. L. Allen, J. L. Cranford, and N. Pay, 1996, *Journal of the American Academy of Audiology, 7*, pp. 282–288.

nique allows a very detailed three-dimensional view (pictures are taken in axial layers similar to CAT scans) of the structure of the normal brain, and the lesions or other forms of pathology that may be present. The MRI, however, while allowing exquisitely detailed views of anatomical structure, is an event fixed at one point in time that provides no clues related to function. This limitation, however, may change in the not too distant future. Before getting to this exciting new development in neuroimaging, the author must first set the stage by describing another relatively new procedure that allows the neuroscientist to view which particular parts of the brain are "working" when its owner is engaged in some kind of behavioral activity.

This technique is called positron emitted tomography (PET scans). When a part of the brain becomes active (goes to work), it requires more energy to do its job. The brain area will need to take in more nutrition to fuel its increased activity. With PET scans, the neuroscientist injects glucose into a major artery (like the carotid artery). If a region of the brain becomes active the glucose will travel to that region to feed it. Before injecting the glucose into the patient, the scientist mixes it with a small portion of fluid that contains radioactive isotopes. This fluid serves as a radioactive tracer that constantly emits gamma rays that can be picked up and recorded by the PET scan equipment. The PET scanner, thus, can trace where the labeled glucose goes and distinguish areas of the brain that are more or less busy at the time. If the patient is looking at pictures, the visual areas of the cortex will "light up" indicating they are working; if sound is presented to the ears, the auditory cortical areas will light up. It is very interesting that patients with schizophrenia, who are exhibiting visual forms of hallucinations, will show increased activity in the visual areas of the brain the same way they would if they were seeing the real thing. The brains of these patients are acting as if they really are seeing things.

In the last few years, neuroscientists have begun to develop ways of combining MRI and PET scans into a single test system that allows obtaining both functional and anatomical information on the same patients. This exciting new tool is called functional MRI (fMRI). This technique promises to open the door for scientists to be able to see exactly where in the complex structure of the brain specific forms of neural function are occurring. If this promise comes to fruition, it will be especially beneficial for all of the behavioral neurosciences, including audiology and speech-language pathology. The fMRI technique involves performing MRI testing at the same time that PET scans are being performed. The regions of the brain that receive increased flows of the radioactive labeled glucose are literally plotted out on top of the detailed underlying anatomical structures that have been revealed by the MRI procedure. At the present time, fMRI is a very expensive procedure and is only being performed at a few medical research centers around the world. As the technique becomes less expensive and more sensitive (revealing greater and greater detail of functional anatomical areas), it will constitute a major boon for our own communication disorders professions. In the years to come, the practicing SLP will likely see more and more reports of fMRI testing included in audiological evaluation reports.

References and Suggestions for Further Reading

In addition to a number of excellent Web sites on the brain that the reader could look at (which will not be listed as they may not remain on line long enough), the author recommends the following published (and probably more permanent) sources that provide a good overview/introduction to the topics covered in the present chapter.

Allen, R. L., Cranford, J. L., & Pay, N. (1996). Central auditory processing in an adult with congenital absence of left temporal lobe. *Journal of the American Academy of Audiology, 7,* 282–288.

Bhatnager, S. C., & Andy, O. J. (1995). Neuroscience for the study of communication disorders. In *Diagnostic techniques and neurological concepts* (pp. 314–331). Baltimore: Williams & Wilkins.

Jerome, K. B. (2003). *Understanding the brain.* National Geographics Books.

Metter, E. J., & Hanson, W. R. (1985). Brain imaging related to speech and language. In J. Darley (Ed.), *Speech evaluation in neurology* (pp.). New York: Grune and Stratton.

Swerdlow, J. L. (1995, June). Quiet miracles of the brain. *National Geographic Magazine, 187*(6), 2–41.

Index

Note: Page numbers in **bold** type reference figures and tables.